Transanal Endoscopic Microsurgery

Peter A. Cataldo · Gerhard F. Buess
Editors

Transanal Endoscopic Microsurgery

Principles and Techniques

Foreword by David J. Schoetz, Jr.

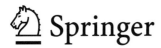

Editors

Peter A. Cataldo
University of Vermont
 College of Medicine
Burlington, VT, USA

Gerhard F. Buess
Eberhard Karls Universitaet
 Tuebingen
Tuebingen, Germany

ISBN: 978-0-387-76397-2   e-ISBN: 978-0-387-76398-9
DOI 10.1007/978-0-387-76397-2

Library of Congress Control Number: 2008936555

© 2009 Springer Science+Business Media, LLC
All rights reserved. This work may not be translated or copied in whole or in part without the written permission of the publisher (Springer Science+Business Media, LLC, 233 Spring Street, New York, NY 10013, USA), except for brief excerpts in connection with reviews or scholarly analysis. Use in connection with any form of information storage and retrieval, electronic adaptation, computer software, or by similar or dissimilar methodology now known or hereafter developed is forbidden.
The use in this publication of trade names, trademarks, service marks, and similar terms, even if they are not identified as such, is not to be taken as an expression of opinion as to whether or not they are subject to proprietary rights.
While the advice and information in this book are believed to be true and accurate at the date of going to press, neither the authors nor the editors nor the publisher can accept any legal responsibility for any errors or omissions that may be made. The publisher makes no warranty, express or implied, with respect to the material contained herein

Printed on acid-free paper

springer.com

I would like to dedicate this book to my family: To my mother, Anne Cataldo, who has taught me I can do anything if I put my mind to it, and to the memory of my father, Felix G. Cataldo, who continues to inspire me; to my wife, Eileen, and my daughters, Colleen and Anna, the reasons I wake up every morning. One final thanks to all my patients who challenge me, inspire me, and bring me satisfaction and gratification beyond measure.

Peter A. Cataldo

Foreword

Cancer of the rectum continues to be a significant health problem in industrialized countries around the world. Relative 5-year survival rates in the USA for cancer of the rectum from 1995 to 2001 improved to 65%, a 15% improvement over 20 years (American Cancer Society, 2007). The reasons for this dramatic improvement include more accurate preoperative staging, aggressive neoadjuvant therapy and improved surgical technique as well as specialty-trained surgeons.

Despite advances in nonoperative techniques of radiation therapy, chemotherapy and immunotherapy, surgical extirpation continues to be the cornerstone of curative treatment of this potentially lethal disease. Radical cancer excision with total mesorectal excision has become the preferred surgical procedure for even early-stage cancers of the rectum. Over the past decade the enthusiasm for local excision (and other local treatments) has given way to persuasive (predominantly retrospective) evidence that the incidence of locoregional recurrence due to unsuspected lymphatic metastases and positive lateral margins is unacceptably high even for stage T_1 tumors. Vigorous attempts to find characteristics of the tumor that would allow successful local treatments are ongoing.

Transanal endoscopic microsurgery (TEM) is a technique for the performance of local excision by way of a binocular magnified operating system developed in the early 1980s. Adoption of the technique was slow, due in part to the complexity of the operative procedure as well as the expense of the equipment. Early adopters of the procedure were few in number. As laparoscopic surgery became more widespread, basic ability to work from a flat screen in relatively small spaces became more commonplace and TEM seemed more feasible. More and more units around the world purchased the equipment and applied the techniques of TEM, particularly in patients with distal rectal cancers for whom radical cancer excision represented the creation of a permanent colostomy.

Peter Cataldo has collected contributions from internationally recognized experts in TEM as well as local excision of rectal cancer. Beginning with a frank discussion of the broad indications and potential problems with TEM, the book then presents a comprehensive pictorial atlas of equipment and setup and a candid presentation of how to get started with the procedure. Complications do occur and are frankly presented.

When one starts doing TEM, the most striking improvement over conventional local excision is the magnification and optical resolution that must result in a better local procedure. Repeatedly, this observation is made by the contributors to this book. One author presents a local recurrence rate for TEM in stage T_1 and T_2 cancers of 0%. All of the published comparative trials demonstrate significantly better oncologic results for rectal cancer treated by TEM than by conventional local excision.

Of interest is the fact that TEM has finally been adopted by the colorectal surgical community at the same time as the current majority opinion is that radical cancer excision is much preferred for distal rectal cancer. Clearly, all of the returns regarding treatment of distal rectal cancer are not in and much of what we do now will change in the near term as techniques evolve.

Not surprisingly, creative individuals have applied TEM for other indications, including benign rectal lesions, complex fistulas and rectourethral and rectovaginal fistulas and even natural orifice transluminal endoscopic surgery (NOTES). As expertise and applications expand, the only limit to the use of this technology (and subsequent improvements) is the imagination of the users.

To my knowledge, this volume represents the first comprehensive description of TEM; it is succinct yet comprehensive and will be a necessary partner in the development and application of this relatively newly discovered procedure.

David J. Schoetz, Jr.
Professor of Surgery
Tufts University School of Medicine
Boston, MA, USA
Lahey Clinic
Burlington, MA, USA

Preface

Transanal endoscopic microsurgery (TEM) was developed in the early 1980s in Tübingen, Germany, by Gerhard Buess and the Richard Wolf Medical Instrument Company to remove large rectal polyps beyond the reach of standard transanal excision. It has blossomed into a valuable, state-of-the-art technology equal to any other technique in terms of reliably positive patient outcome. Its role has expanded beyond excision of colonoscopically unresectable polyps to include removal of select, early rectal cancers with or without adjuvant chemoradiation therapy, the treatment of anastomotic strictures, and repair of proximal, complex rectal fistulae. TEM was initially embraced more rapidly in Europe (particularly Germany and Italy), but is now becoming well established in the USA and Canada. TEM has been embraced by many of the leading teaching hospitals and highly respected colon and rectal clinics throughout the USA. The number of cases performed each year is increasing substantially, with an estimated 800 performed in 2007.

Transanal Endoscopic Microsurgery: Principals and Techniques is the first and only book solely dedicated to TEM and we are hopeful it will become the standard reference for the technique. It is our hope that the book will be well received and widely read so that all patients who can benefit from this technique will have that opportunity. Expert authors from around the world have dedicated their precious time and created outstanding chapters on all aspects of TEM. Special thanks to each of them. Gerhard Buess, the father and inventor of TEM, has worked countless hours creating an incredibly detailed DVD with outstanding video clips that clearly and beautifully demonstrate all the important technical aspects of this challenging procedure. He has been and continues to be a mentor to me and many other TEM surgeons. We are all profoundly grateful.

In addition, Tina Blais-Armell has worked tirelessly, without complaint, and with little thanks to coordinate the efforts of all involved; without her there would be no book. I owe her a great debt of thanks. Paula Callaghan and Lindsey Reilly from Springer have provided much needed help in moving this project along, prodding those who needed prodding and doing all the little things no one notices—thank you Paula and Lindsey!

Peter A. Cataldo

Contents

Foreword... vii
Preface.. ix
Contributors... xiii

1 Indications.. 1
Mark H. Whiteford

2 Preoperative Preparation.................................... 7
Garnet J. Blatchford and N. Anh Tran

3 Equipment and Operative Set-up............................. 13
Lee E. Smith

**4 Pelvic Anatomic Considerations for Transanal Endoscopic
Microsurgery**... 27
Peter A. Cataldo

5 Getting Started.. 35
Patricia L. Roberts

6 Partial-Thickness Excision.................................. 41
Peter A. Cataldo and Neil J. Mortensen

7 Full-Thickness Excision.................................... 47
Emanuele Lezoche, Mario Guerrieri,
Maddalena Baldarelli and Giovanni Lezoche

8 Advanced Surgical Techniques............................... 59
Prakash Gatta and Lee L. Swanstrom

9 Complications.. 75
K.S. Khanduja

10 Comparison with Traditional Techniques...................... 85
Matthew R. Dixon and Charles O. Finne

| 11 | **Full-Thickness Local Excision** | 109 |
| | Lauren A. Kosinski, John H. Marks, and Gerald J. Marks | |

| 12 | **Oncologic Outcomes** | 117 |
| | Joel E. Goldberg and Ronald Bleday | |

| 13 | **Clinical Trials** | 125 |
| | Kim F. Rhoads and Julio E. Garcia-Aguilar | |

| 14 | **Future Directions** | 135 |
| | Mark Choh and Theodore J. Saclarides | |

Index 141

Contributors

Maddalena Baldarelli, MD
Clinica di Chirurgia Generale e Metodologia Chirurgica, Università Politecnica delle Marche, Ospedali Riuniti di Ancona, Ancona, Italy

Garnet J. Blatchford, MD
Creighton University, Omaha, NE, University of Nebraska Medical Center, Omaha, NE, USA

Ronald Bleday, MD
Section of Colorectal Surgery, Brigham and Women's Hospital, Harvard Medical School, Boston, MA, USA

Gerhard F. Buess, MD, FRCS
Eberhard Karls Universitaet Tuebingen, Tuebingen, Germany

Peter A. Cataldo, MD, FACS, FASCRS
University of Vermont College of Medicine, Burlington, VT, USA

Mark Choh, MD
Rush Medical College, Rush University Medical Center, Chicago, IL, USA

Matthew R. Dixon, MD
Department of Surgery, Kaiser Permanente, Oakland, CA, USA

Charles O. Finne, MD
University of Minnesota, Minneapolis, MN, USA

Prakash Gatta, MBBS
Department of Surgery, University Hospital, University of Cincinnati, Cincinnati, OH, USA

Julio E. Garcia-Aguilar, MD
University of California, San Francisco, San Francisco, CA, USA

Joel E. Goldberg, MD
Brigham and Women's Hospital, Harvard Medical School, Boston, MA, USA

Mario Guerrieri, MD
Clinica di Chirurgia Generale e Metodologia Chirurgica, Università Politecnica delle Marche, Ospedali Riuniti di Ancona, Ancona, Italy

K.S. Khanduja, MD, FACS, FASCRS
Mount Carmel Health System, The Ohio State University Medical Center, Columbus, OH, USA

Lauren A. Kosinski, MD, MS
Lankenau, Bryn Mawr, and Paoli Hospitals, Wynnewood, PA, USA

Emanuele Lezoche, MD
Dipartimento di Chirurgia Paride Stefanini, La Sapienza Universita' Di Roma, Policlinico Umberto I, Rome, Italy

Giovanni Lezoche
Dipartimento di Chirurgia Paride Stefanini, La Sapienza Universita' Di Roma, Policlinico Umberto I, Rome, Italy

Gerald J. Marks, MD
Drexel University, Philadelphia, PA, Marks Colorectal Surgical Associates, Lankenau Hospital, Wynnewood, PA, USA

John H. Marks, MD
Lankenau, Bryn Mawr, and Paoli Hospitals, Wynnewood, PA, USA

Neil J. Mortensen, MD, FR
John Radcliffe Hospital, Oxford, UK

Kim F. Rhoads, MD, MS, MPH
Mt. Zion Cancer Center, University of California, San Francisco, San Francisco, CA, USA

Patricia L. Roberts, MD
Tufts University School of Medicine, Boston, MA, Lahey Clinic, Burlington, MA, USA

Theodore J. Saclarides, MD
Rush Medical College, Rush University Medical Center, Chicago, IL, USA

Lee E. Smith, MD, FACS
Georgetown University, Colon and Rectal Surgery, Washington Hospital Center, Washington, DC, USA

Lee L. Swanstrom, MD
Minimally Invasive Surgery, Legacy Health System and Oregon Clinic, Portland, OR, USA

N. Anh Tran, MD
Creighton University Medical Center, Omaha, NE, USA

Mark H. Whiteford, MD, FACS, FASCRS
Oregon Health and Science University, Legacy Portland Hospitals, Portland, OR, USA

Chapter 1
Indications

Mark H. Whiteford

Transanal techniques have long been used for management of rectal diseases. Transanal local excision of rectal tumors was popularized by Parks et al. in the 1950s and is well suited for the management of selected low rectal lesions. Removal of lesions in the middle and upper rectum presents a more challenging problem owing to the limited accessibility and inadequate exposure afforded by standard instrumentation. These more proximal lesions have traditionally been managed by low anterior, abdominoperineal, transsacral, and transsphincteric resections. The transanal endoscopic microsurgery (TEM) operating system now offers a low morbidity and often outpatient alternative to these more radical surgical options.

TEM allows greater versatility and options for the operating surgeon. In addition to extending the surgeon's reach up to the distal sigmoid colon, the four ports of access allow for synchronous use of an illuminated camera, forceps, cautery, suction as well as the freedom to use common laparoscopic techniques such as suturing, ultrasonic dissectors, and bipolar and other energy sources.

TEM is used to treat a variety of disease processes, both benign and malignant. Table 1.1 illustrates the diverse indications reported in several large series and registries. Still others have described repair of high supralevator fistulas, rectourethral fistulas, drainage of pelvic collections, and excision of extrarectal masses [3, 7]. By far, the most common uses of TEM are for resection of colonoscopically unresectable rectal adenomas and carefully selected rectal cancers. It should be stressed that even though TEM extends the reach of conventional transanal resections, it should not change the stringent indications for resection, especially in regard to rectal cancer.

Resection of rectal and distal sigmoid adenomas is the most appealing indication for TEM. These are benign lesions in which patients can be spared the morbidity of an unnecessary mesorectal dissection. Smaller adenomas without evidence of high-grade dysplasia may be removed by submucosal dissection. Larger adenomas or those with high-grade dysplasia are at high risk of harboring invasive adenocarcinoma and should be excised full thickness with a 10-mm resection margin. Still others recommend full-thickness resection with en bloc removal of the adjacent mesorectum when resecting cancer with curative intent [8]. When there is suspicion but not confirmation of a malignant rectal polyp in a patient unfit for or unwilling to undergo major abdominal surgery, TEM can be useful in resecting the entire lesion in one piece for complete histologic assessment. Prompt radical surgery, if indicated, can be performed without significantly increasing morbidity.

M.H. Whiteford (✉)
Oregon Health and Science University, Legacy Portland Hospitals, Portland, OR, USA

P.A. Cataldo, G.F. Buess (eds.), *Transanal Endoscopic Microsurgery*,
DOI 10.1007/978-0-387-76397-2_1, © Springer Science+Business Media, LLC 2009

Table 1.1 Indications for transanal endoscopic microsurgery reported by disease process

	Salm et al. [1]	Smith et al. [2]	Steele et al. [3]	Mentges et al. [4]	Saclarides [5]	Palma et al. [6]
Adenoma	1,411	82	77	236	28	71
Carcinoma	435	54	23	98	43	23
Carcinoid		5		7	2	5
Rectal prolapse	22	1		7		1
Rectal ulcer		1		2		
Non-Hodgkin's lymphoma				1		
Angiodysplasia				1		
Diverticulum				1		
Epithelioid cell granuloma				1		
Hyperplastic polyp				1		
Stricture		3				
Rectal stump excision		1				
Endometrioma		3				
Enterovaginal fistula		2				

TEM may also be useful as a palliative tool in patients with extensive metastatic disease or those medically unfit to withstand radical surgery. Neoadjuvant radiation therapy, when used in conjunction with resection either for cure or palliation, does not appear to increase complications following TEM [8].

The limited access and visibility afforded by traditional transanal retractors has restricted their use to resection of rectal polyps and cancers which are mobile, less than 8–10 cm from the anal verge, are smaller than 3–4 cm, and occupy less than 40% of the rectal circumference [9, 10]. The TEM technique permits access to the entire rectum, including lesions with a proximal margin located 20 cm from the anal verge. Resections of larger or more proximal lesions are technically more demanding, but with experience, these, as well as circumferential sleeve resections, can be performed safely [4, 11].

The inferior limit for effective use of the TEM instrument is the upper anal canal, approximately 3–4 cm proximal to the anal verge. When the surgeon is operating this low, the aperture of the operating proctoscope is prone to slipping downward and out of the anal canal. This results in escape of the CO_2 pneumorectum, collapse of the operative field, and loss of adequate exposure of the target lesion. Low rectal lesions, however, are good opportunities for surgeons to gain TEM operative experience, for if the TEM experience does not proceed as planned, excision can be performed with conventional transanal techniques [11]. The TEM learning experience and confidence should first be gained operating on small, distal lesions with subsequent progression to larger then more proximal lesions. Most resections can be performed through the shorter (120-mm-length) proctoscope. The longer (200-mm) TEM proctoscope has reduced degrees of freedom for instruments, is more prone to instrument conflict, and therefore is harder for the novice to operate through than the shorter proctoscope.

Resection of anterior rectal lesions requires special attention. Full-thickness excision of the anterior and even lateral rectum carries the risk of inadvertent dissection into the vagina, urethra, or bladder. Failure of adequate closure may lead to a rectourethral or rectovaginal fistula. There is little mention of this complication in the literature, suggesting its occurrence is rare.

Table 1.2 Average mean anterior, lateral, and posterior length measurements from the anal verge to the peritoneal reflection. (From Table 3 in Najarian et al. [12] with kind permission of Springer Science+ Business Media)

	Women	Men	p
Anterior (cm)	9 (5.5–13.5)	9.7 (7–16)	NS
Lateral (cm)	12.2 (8.5–17)	12.8 (9–19)	NS
Posterior (cm)	14.8 (11–19)	15.5 (12–20)	NS

Ranges are in *parentheses*.
NS not significant.

In an interesting in vitro anatomical study, Najarian et al. [12] documented the mean distance from the anal verge to peritoneal reflection (Table 1.2). This information should be considered in preoperative planning for TEM as intraperitoneal access, while unusual, may occur during full-thickness resection of more proximal rectal lesions.

Intraperitoneal entry carries a risk of injuring intraabdominal structures, bacterial and potential cytologic contamination, and anastomotic leak. Initially regarded as a complication, with experience, intraperitoneal excision with secure closure of the rectal defect can be performed without increased short-term morbidity [13]. If there is concern about the adequacy of an intraperitoneal closure, the patient may be observed overnight for signs of a leak and undergo a water-soluble contrast enema the following morning.

Bulky lesions such as large pedunculated or circumferential polyps can be challenging to manage with any transanal technique, including TEM. These larger specimens can be difficult to see around and are prone to fragmentation and bleeding. Hemorrhage under these circumstances may be particularly difficult to isolate and control. Fragmentation may theoretically lead to cytologic dissemination and increased recurrence rates.

Colorectal anastomotic and short postinflammatory strictures are infrequent occurrences but are particularly amenable to endoscopic management. Most published reports describe colonoscopic management in combination with pneumatic dilatation, Nd:YAG laser, argon beam coagulation, or electrocautery stricturoplasty [14–16]. There are also reports of transanal stricturoplasty using an operating urologic rectoscope [17]. There is a paucity of similar reports on the use of these techniques in combination with the TEM equipment [2, 18]. Nonetheless, this would be an appropriate indication for TEM provided the stricture is 5–15 cm from the anal verge. Strictures less than 5 cm from the anal verge will not allow insertion of the 40-mm-diameter TEM proctoscope.

Contraindications for TEM are few. These include patients unfit for general or regional anesthesia, uncorrected coagulopathy, rectal varicies, and anal stenosis. A careful history of prior surgery with pelvic mesh placement should also be sought as this may hinder access of the operating proctoscope. Caution should also be taken in patients with a remote history of high-dose pelvic radiation therapy for gynecologic or urologic malignancies. Chronic radiation-induced changes are known to predispose patients to decreased rectal compliance, stenosis, friability, and impaired wound healing.

The surgeon's personal skills and experience will also determine some of the limitations of TEM. The disease processes treated by TEM, namely, colonoscopically unresectable rectal polyps and early cancers, are far less common in clinical practice than those disease processes treated by abdominal laparoscopic operations. This limits any single surgeon's or institution's volume and operative experience. The TEM instrumentation can lead to a variety of new challenges for operating surgeons. Long, modified laparoscopic instruments are introduced and manipulated in a parallel fashion through a narrow proctoscope. This can lead to instrument conflict, difficult tissue exposure, suboptimal traction and counter-traction, and the technical hurdle of suturing closed a transverse defect using longitudinally oriented instruments.

Several factors have caused a rebirth of enthusiasm for TEM in the USA and abroad. First is the recently rekindled controversy surrounding increased local recurrence rates following standard transanal resection of favorable early rectal cancers. TEM offers some theoretic advantages over standard transanal excision of neoplasms. These include better visualization of the surgical field and tumor margins, gentler tissue handling with potentially less tumor fragmentation and dissemination, and better ability to perform an en bloc resection of the adjacent, potentially tumor bearing, mesorectum [8, 19]. Second, more and more surgeons are being trained with advanced, two-handed, laparoscopic skills. These skills are required to be facile with and take full advantage of the TEM equipment, advance through the learning curve, and not succumb to frustration, which can lead to abandonment of the technique.

The future may reveal a third potential use of TEM as a portal to the peritoneum for natural orifice translumenal endoscopic surgery (NOTES). Transgastric endoscopic peritonoscopy, cholecystectomy, appendectomy, and tubal ligation are now active areas of basic science and clinical research. Transrectal (or transvaginal) access to the peritoneum via TEM may permit application of larger, more versatile instruments, removal of larger organs, maintenance of pneumoperitoneum, in-line instead of retroflexed views of upper abdominal organs, and secure suture closure of the proctotomy. The Society of American Gastrointestinal and Endoscopic Surgeons (SAGES) and the American Society for Gastrointestinal Endoscopy (ASGE) have collaborated to form a NOTES working group and the Natural Orifice Surgery Consortium for Assessment and Research (NOSCAR) in an effort to facilitate research and safe clinical introduction of this emerging field [20].

References

1. Salm R, Lampe H, Bustos A, Matern U. Experience with TEM in Germany. *Endosc Surg Allied Technol* 1994;2:251–54.
2. Smith LE, Ko ST, Saclarides T, Caushaj P, Orkin BA, Khanduja KS. Transanal endoscopic microsurgery. Initial Registry Results. *Dis Colon Rectum* 1996;39:S79–S84.
3. Steele RJC, Hershman MJ, Mortensen NJ, Armitage NCM, Scholefield JH. Transanal endoscopic microsurgery-initial experience from three centres in the United Kingdom. *Br J Surg* 1996;83:207–210.
4. Mentges B, Buess G, Schafer D, Manncke K, Becker HD. Local therapy for rectal tumours. *Dis Colon Rectum.* 1996;39:886–92.
5. Saclarides TJ. Transanal Endoscopic Microsurgery: A single surgeon's experience. *Arch Surg* 1998;133:595–98.
6. Palma P, Freudenberg S, Samel S, Post S. Transanal endoscopic microsurgery: indications and results after 100 cases. *Colorectal Dis* 2004;6:350–5.
7. Cataldo PA. Transanal endoscopic microsurgery. *Surg Clin N Am* 2006;86:915–25.
8. Lezoche E, Guerrieri M, Paganini AM, D'Ambrosio G, Baldarelli M, Lezoche G, Feliciotti F, DeSanctis A. Transanal endoscopic vs total mesorectal laparoscopic resections of T2-N0 low rectal cancers after neoadjuvant treatment: a prospective randomized trial with a 3-year minimum follow-up period. *Surg Endosc* 2005;19:751–756.
9. Steele GD, Herndon JE, Bleday R, Russell A, Benson A, Hussain M, Burgess A, Tepper JE, Mayer RJ. Sphincter-sparing treatment for distal rectal adenocarcinoma. *Ann Surg Onc* 1999;6:433–41.
10. Corman, ML. Carcinoma of the rectum. In: Colon and Rectal Surgery, 5th edition. Corman ML, ed. Phiadelphia: Lippincott Williams &Wilkins, 2005:905–1061.
11. Saclarides TJ, Smith L, Ko ST, Orkin B, Buess G. Transanal endoscopic microsurgery. *Dis Colon Rectum* 1992;35:1183–1191.

1 Indications

12. Najarian MM, Belzer GE, Cogbill TH, Mathiason MA. Determination of the peritoneal reflection using intraoperative proctoscopy. *Dis Colon Rectum* 2004;47:2080–2085.
13. Gavagan JA, Whiteford MH, Swanstrom LL. Full thickness intraperitoneal excision by transanal endoscopic microsurgery does not increase short-term complications. *Am J Surg* 2004;187:630–34.
14. Luchtefeld MA, Milsom JW, Senagore A, Surrell JA, Maxier WP Colorectal anastomotic stenosis: results of a survey of the ASCRS Membership. *Dis Colon Rectum* 1989;32:733–736.
15. Brandimarte G, Tursi A, Gasbarrini G. Endoscopic treatment of benign anastomotic colorectal stenosis with electrocautery. *Endoscopy* 2000;32:461–3.
16. Suchan KL, Muldner A, Manegold BC. Endoscopic treatment of postoperative colorectal anastomotic strictures. *Surg Endosc* 2003;17:1110–3.
17. Hunt TM, Kelly MJ. Endoscopic transanal resection (ETAR) of colorectal strictures in stapled anastomoses. *Ann R Coll Surg Engl* 1994;76:121–2
18. Kato K, Saito T, Matsuda M, Imai M, Kasai S, Mito M. Successful treatment of a rectal anastomotic stenosis by transanal endoscopic microsurgery (TEM) using the contact Nd:YAG laser. *Surg Endosc* 1997;11:485–87.
19. Floyd ND, Saclarides TJ. Transanal endoscopic microsurgical resection of pT1 rectal tumors. *Dis Colon Rectum* 2005;49:164–8.
20. ASGE/SAGES Working group on Natural Orifice Translumenal Endoscopic Surgery. White Paper. October 2005. *Gastrointest Endosc* 2006;63:199–203.

Chapter 2
Preoperative Preparation

Garnet J. Blatchford and N. Anh Tran

Transanal endoscopic microsurgery (TEM) is a technique which offers exceptionally good visualization combined with the ability to precisely excise lesions throughout the rectum. One of the greatest advantages of TEM excision is that even large lesions can be removed intact and both deep and radial margins can be assessed. TEM requires careful preoperative preparation in order to avoid complications and maximize patient benefits.

Consent

Informed consent for TEM should include a discussion about the nature of the procedure and its potential risks and complications. These include, but are not limited to, incontinence, bleeding, perforation, rectovaginal fistula, incomplete resection, and inability to resect the lesion. Our approach has been to inform patients the TEM equipment provides us with the ability to do an excisional or "superbiopsy" of the lesion. It should be made clear to the patients that this may be only the first step in the diagnosis of their problem and they may require further surgery to complete their treatment.

Owing to the size of the TEM scope (4-cm diameter), there is some anal dilation which occurs in most patients during the procedure, and they may experience short-term incontinence postoperatively [1]. A significant number of patients have preoperative incontinence, and this should be documented. Fortunately, long-term incontinence after TEM is rare and much less frequent than following a low anterior resection.

Significant bleeding may occur with either submucosal or full-thickness excision. This can develop during the procedure or up to several weeks postoperatively. Such bleeding may require further endoscopic treatment or even radical surgery, although this is very uncommon. Nonsteroidals and other anticoagulants may need to be stopped 1–2 weeks prior to surgery.

Full-thickness resection of the rectum can result in inadvertent entry into the vagina or peritoneal cavity. This is more common in anterior lesions in the upper rectum, particularly in women who have had a hysterectomy. Suture closure may be performed; however, leak and abscess may result. Depending on the extent of resection and success of closure, laparoscopic inspection or formal resection may be required [2]. Some surgeons advocate obtaining consent for formal celiotomy and resection along with the TEM consent, but we do not do this routinely.

G.J. Blatchford (✉)
Creighton University, Omaha, NE, University of Nebraska Medical Center, Omaha, NE, USA

P.A. Cataldo, G.F. Buess (eds.), *Transanal Endoscopic Microsurgery*,
DOI 10.1007/978-0-387-76397-2_2, © Springer Science+Business Media, LLC 2009

A discussion should be held with the patient who has an upper rectal lesion regarding options should the lesion not be amenable to TEM excision. Risk of incomplete removal or inaccessibility is increased with proximal rectal lesions owing to the angulation and narrow lumen at this level. Alternatives might include piecemeal polypectomy or formal resection depending on the individual situation, and this can be done at the same time or at a later date.

Evaluation of the Lesion

Full colonic evaluation should be done preoperatively to identify any synchronous lesions. Most rectal lesions should be examined by endorectal ultrasound to determine the depth of penetration into the rectal wall. In addition, endorectal ultrasound can detect the presence of suspicious lymph nodes, a contraindication to TEM for cure of malignant lesions. Endorectal ultrasound has accuracy for depth of invasion from 75 to 90% and can be used to identify patients with T_2 lesions who may require adjuvant chemoradiotherapy, and T_3 lesions not appropriate for curative TEM. If the ultrasound suggests that a large lesion is completely confined to the mucosa, then dissection in the submucosal plane is sufficient. Ultrasound for large polyps may be more accurate than endoscopic biopsy to identify an occult invasive cancer [3]. Similarly, if there is a suggestion of invasion deep to the submucosa on ultrasound (even in the face of endoscopic biopsies giving negative findings) then a full-thickness excision should be performed.

Exact localization (both height and orientation) of the lesion by rigid proctoscopy in the preoperative period is essential prior to TEM excision. Measurement of the level of the lesion by flexible endoscopy is notoriously unreliable. Proctoscopy will reveal the exact distance from the dentate line. Lesions just above the dentate line may be easier to remove without TEM since carbon dioxide may escape, resulting in inadequate distention of the rectum if the scope is positioned too low. In addition, lesions above the 15-cm region may not be amenable to TEM excision if the rectoscope diameter exceeds the diameter of the rectosigmoid, precluding the passage of the scope to the necessary level. In this situation, consent for low anterior resection may be obtained preoperatively if complete TEM excision is deemed impossible. Finally, the correct orientation of the lesion anteriorly, posteriorly, or laterally is best determined by rigid proctoscopy, and this will have important implications in positioning the patient for the TEM procedure. Ideally, the lesion must be placed down in order to facilitate ease of TEM excision. Consequently, an anterior lesion will require a prone position, and conversely, a posterior lesion will require a lithotomy position. When a larger lesion encompasses a significant portion of the circumference, it may be necessary to remove part of the lesion and then change the position of the patient to facilitate removal of the remaining portion.

Preparation of the Lesion

In order to facilitate TEM excision of a lesion, it is sometimes necessary to manipulate the lesion itself preoperatively. This might include tattooing of the site or debulking of the lesion. The timing of these techniques will depend a lot on the nature of the lesion itself. Timing of TEM excision from the original polypectomy at colonoscopy can be crucial. If done too soon, dissection planes will be distorted from the inflammation secondary to the polypectomy itself. If TEM excision proceeds too late, the polypectomy site can be completely healed, making identification of the site difficult or impossible.

Tattooing is important if a small lesion has been removed and further excision is warranted. Such a situation can arise if polypectomy during colonoscopy results in a pathologic diagnosis of carcinoid or adenocarcinoma with questionable margins. Since this finding will likely have been unsuspected at the time of the colonoscopy, the polypectomy site could heal and potentially become unidentifiable in the near future, particularly if there is a delay between diagnosis and referral to the surgeon. This becomes especially pertinent if TEM cannot be scheduled expeditiously. A tattoo in the area is useful to direct further excision. Patients should be brought back for tattooing as soon as possible. Once they have been tattooed, further excision can be scheduled at a more leisurely pace. Ideally, the surgeon who will perform the TEM excision should do the tattooing so the India ink can be placed appropriately. An indiscriminate tattoo at the site can make TEM excision more difficult, turning all the tissue black and making the planes difficult to see. The preferred technique is to inject circumferentially a short distance away from the lesion, preferably at the margin of excision. This leaves an "outline" around the lesion, but no ink left within the actual lesion site itself. Injections should be in the submucosal plane and not mucosa as the mucosa will rapidly turn over, causing the tattoo to disappear.

Large bulky polyps may be easier to remove by TEM if the protuberant portion of the polyp is snared prior to the TEM procedure. If not, the polyp may prolapse into the rectoscope, making visualization of the base of the lesion tricky. Debulking can be done at the time of the original colonoscopy if further TEM excision is contemplated, or it can be done intraoperatively just prior to excision. In addition to the usual TEM equipment, one would only need a wire snare (either a proctoscopic or flexible endoscopic snare). This is manipulated through the port of TEM faceplate. Graspers can be used to assist in placement of the snare. An advantage of debulking on the day of surgery is that there will be minimal to no distortion of the tissue planes secondary to inflammation caused by polypectomy.

Bowel Preparation

Recently, many studies have questioned the need for a mechanical bowel preparation even for abdominal bowel resections. Controversy still exists regarding the necessity of bowel cleansing as some authors have concluded that outcomes are similar for those who undergo a bowel preparation and those who do not. The variety of cathartics, enemas, and lavages available multiplied by the numerous antibiotic regimens can lead to an exponential number of possible combinations for a suitable bowel preparation. These choices can be dizzying, but practice mainly depends on surgeon preference. Most surgeons agree that at least a single-dose systemic antibiotic preoperatively is mandatory.

For TEM excision specifically, bowel preparation may depend on the extent of excision, location of the lesion, and intent of abdominal resection should TEM excision fail. If the lesion is low-lying and excision will be entirely extraperitoneal, some may proceed with a preparation similar to that for hemorrhoidectomy (Fleet enema on the morning of the procedure). However, we prefer a full bowel preparation, especially if there is any possibility of invading the peritoneum during excision. In our practice, this involves both a mechanical preparation of choice (polyethylene glycol or Fleet phosphosoda) in addition to both oral antibiotics (erythromycin and metronidazole) the day prior to surgery and systemic antibiotics (cefotetan) preoperatively. In general, antibiotics do not need to be continued postoperatively.

Deep Venous Thrombosis Prophylaxis

Prevention of venous thromboembolism is the responsibility of every surgeon. It incurs an enormous amount of hospital morbidity and mortality. Without prophylaxis, the incidence of hospital-acquired deep venous thrombosis is 10–40%, and pulmonary embolism accounts for nearly a third of hospital deaths [4]. With this in mind, the surgeon should not shirk his/her duty to ensure adequate prophylaxis.

Although the possibility of venous thromboembolism is not nearly as high in TEM as it is in major abdominal surgery, a definite risk still exists. Because major abdominal surgery is often undesirable in this population, TEM patients tend to skew older with patients who inevitably have more medical comorbidities. Although unlikely, there is also the possibility of occult malignancy. Other factors that can contribute to risk are positioning and length of the procedure. Also, as surgeons begin to learn the technique of TEM, the procedure can last several hours. The risk factors for venous thromboembolism subsequently multiply even for a relatively straightforward procedure such as TEM excision.

In our practice, we institute preoperative prophylaxis with 5,000 units of unfractionated heparin subcutaneously and continue this postoperatively every 8–12 h until discharge. Patients are fitted with support hose and sequential compression devices unless we anticipate a very uncomplicated excision. Even so, we have encountered one patient who suffered bilateral pulmonary embolism postoperatively.

Prevention of Urinary Retention

Urinary retention is a well-known common complication of anorectal surgery. Risk factors include fluid overload, rectal spasm, narcotic pain medicine, and spinal anesthesia. We caution our anesthesiologists on judicious hydration, and often TEM patients will not require narcotic analgesics secondary to the location of the incision (above the dentate line). Most patient discomfort arises from anal dilatation because of the operating proctoscope, and this is usually not severe. It is our practice to straight-catheterize all our patients at the conclusion of the procedure unless the procedure takes less than 1 h. This ensures an empty bladder in recovery and has decreased our rate of urinary retention.

Conclusion

Uncertainty regarding location, orientation, and potential invasion of the lesion will lead to prolonged operative times and possible inadequate treatment. Informed consent prepares the patient for all likely outcomes. Tattooing or debulking of the lesion can facilitate removal. Careful preoperative evaluation, preparation, and planning will expedite the TEM procedure.

References

1. Kreis M, Ekkehard C, Haug V, Manncke K, Buess G. Functional Results After Transanal Endoscopic Microsurgery. Dis Colon Rectum 1996;39:1116–1121.
2. Saclarides T, Smith L, Ko S, Orkin B, Buess G. Transanal Endoscopic Microsurgery. Dis Colon Rectum 1992;35:1183–91.
3. Mentges B, Buess G, Schafer D, Manncke K, Becker H. Local Therapy of Rectal Tumors. Dis Colon Rectum 1996;39:886–892.
4. Geerts W, Pineo G, Heit J, et al. Preventiion of Venous Thromboembolism: The Seventh ACCP Conference on Antithrombotic and Thrombolytic Therapy. Chest 2004;126:338S–400S.

Chapter 3
Equipment and Operative Set-up

Lee E. Smith

The equipment for transanal endoscopic microsurgery (TEM) was designed in the early 1980s well prior to the advent of therapeutic laparoscopy for general surgery, and was developed to overcome the problem of exposure and access to the upper two thirds of the rectum. Owing to the nature of rectal anatomy, the operating proctoscopes and instruments are long and narrow. The insufflation/suction/irrigation machine provides the exposure necessary to carry out the cutting, dissecting, and sewing required. The equipment is fitted with locking gaskets and caps to maintain a gastight system, thus keeping the rectum insufflated to facilitate operative exposure.

Equipment

Articulated Stabilizing Arm

The articulated arm, also known as the Martin arm, attaches to the operating table and serves as a brace to hold the operating proctoscope firmly in place. There are two ball joints which fully articulate and are locked firmly in place with a single set screw. A bar at the one end of the articulated arm attaches to the rail on the operating table using a standard or universal operating table clamp (Fig. 3.1). At the opposite end the articulated arm attaches to the operating proctoscope. The two right angles in the arm permit placement of the double joints upright, beneath the handle of the proctoscope, allowing for secure fixation of the proctoscope without interfering with the surgeon's ability to manipulate the instruments.

Operative Proctoscopes

The operating proctoscope is 4 cm in diameter and is available in two lengths, 12 and 20 cm, and allows for access throughout the rectum (Fig. 3.2). The shaft of the scope is marked in centimeters to allow the surgeon to identify the level of the insertion. The scope shaft locks

---

L.E. Smith (✉)
Georgetown University, Colon and Rectal Surgery, Washington Hospital Center, Washington, DC, USA

P.A. Cataldo, G.F. Buess (eds.), *Transanal Endoscopic Microsurgery*,
DOI 10.1007/978-0-387-76397-2_3, © Springer Science+Business Media, LLC 2009

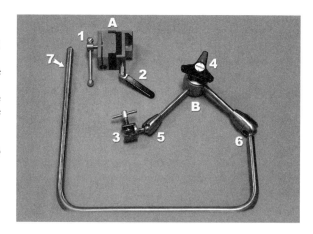

Fig. 3.1 Articulated arm system. *A* universal clamp, *1* the tightening handle for attaching and holding the end of the steel brace to the operating table, *2* tightening handle for attachment of the clamp to the rail of the operating table, *b* articulated arm, *3* clamp for attaching the arm to the handle of the operating proctoscope, *4* the double-ball joint tightening handle, *5, 6* the two ball joints, *7* the end of the steel brace that attaches to the universal clamp

into a rotating collar on the handle, which preserves an airtight seal (Fig. 3.3). This handle has a port to which a hand-bulb insufflator can be attached, or to which a tube is connected for monitoring the CO_2 pressure (Fig. 3.3b).

Two types of faceplate are available and both are routinely used during the conduct of an operation. (Fig. 3.4a, b) Both types are fitted into the handle and locked with an airtight lever. The first type has a clear glass face (Fig. 3.4a), which is used for initial positioning of the scope (similar to rigid proctoscopy). This faceplate is used with a hand-bulb insufflator attached to the port on the handle, which is used to distend the rectal wall, permitting identification of the lesion for proper positioning (Fig. 3.4a). The second type is the operating faceplate (Fig. 3.4b, c). This faceplate has a port for the optics and a snap-on multiport piece (Fig. 3.4c), which contains three ports for the long operating instruments. These ports are covered with airtight caps for maintaining pneumorectum and are fitted with holes, which may be of different sizes, to accommodate instruments of different diameters. The right-side operating port is slightly larger and thus requires a slightly larger cap. Within the snap-on multiport piece are flap valves that serve to help prevent gas leaks (Fig. 3.4c).

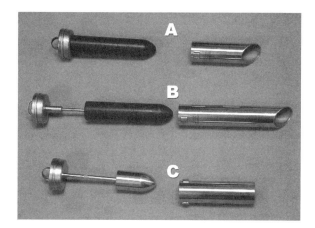

Fig. 3.2 Operating proctoscopes and obturators. *A* 12-cm scope with beveled tip, *B* 20-cm scope with beveled tip, *C* 12-cm scope with flat tip

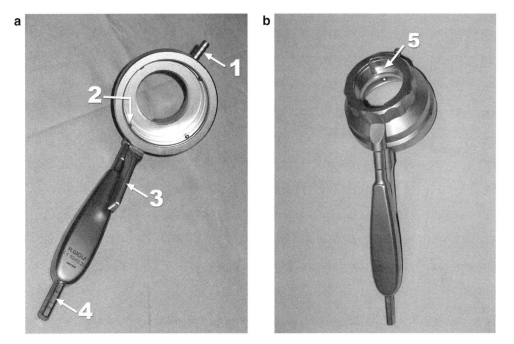

Fig. 3.3 **a** Operating proctoscope handle. *1* port for CO_2 pressure monitoring line or the hand-insufflation bulb, *2* one of the locking pins for attaching the faceplates, *3* the locking handle for the faceplate, *4* rod for engagement of the handle to the clamp at the end of the articulated arm. **b** Operating proctoscope handle. *5* slot in the rotating, locking collar to affix the proctoscope to the handle

Optics

The surgeon uses a 10-mm binocular optic (stereoscope) which provides a high-definition, three-dimensional view (Fig. 3.5a). This optic has a long, rigid shaft that is inserted into the optic port on the faceplate and extends the length of the operating proctoscope (Fig. 3.5b). The light cord is attached to the light post protruding vertically from this shaft. A 40°, 5-mm scope is inserted within the stereoscope and is attached to a laparoscopic camera to allow viewing on a video monitor (Fig. 3.5a). The binocular scope has two ports to which tubing is attached for water and CO_2 insufflation (Fig. 3.5c). The light, binocular optics, water jet, port for monocular optic, and CO_2 converge at the tip within the proctoscope. Each of the optics has a lock to maintain an airtight seal (Fig. 3.5b).

Long Instruments

Long instruments are needed to reach up into the rectum via the operating proctoscopes. The instruments include an electric knife (electrocautery), straight and angled forceps, scissors, suction probe, clip applier, needle holder, and retractable needle (Fig. 3.6a, b).

The long, rigid, high-frequency, electric knife has an angled, pointed tip which is insulated so that only the distal 2–3 mm conducts the electric current. The electrocautery machine is connected to a foot control, which has the alternative of a cutting or cautery

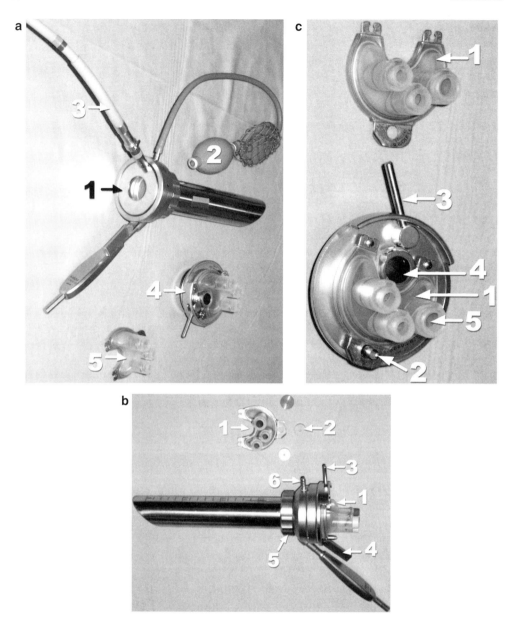

Fig. 3.4 a Operating proctoscope. *1* assembled with the clear-glass faceplate, *2* hand-insufflation bulb, *3* light cord, *4* operating faceplate with the clip-on multiport piece, *5* clip-on multiport piece. **b** Operating proctoscope. *1* clip-on multiport face piece, *2* cap for attachment to the port (note the hole in the cap for introduction of instruments), *3* lock for fixing the binocular stereoscope, *4* lock for the faceplate, *5* locking collar for connecting the handle to the scope, *6* port for the CO_2 pressure monitoring tube or the hand-insufflation bulb. **c** Operating faceplate. *1* the clip-on multiport face piece, *2* clip for attaching the base of the multiport piece, *3* lock for the binocular stereoscope, *4* opening for the introduction of the binocular stereoscope, *5* flap valve within one of the ports to minimize gas loss when an instrument is introduced or removed

3 Equipment and Operative Set-up

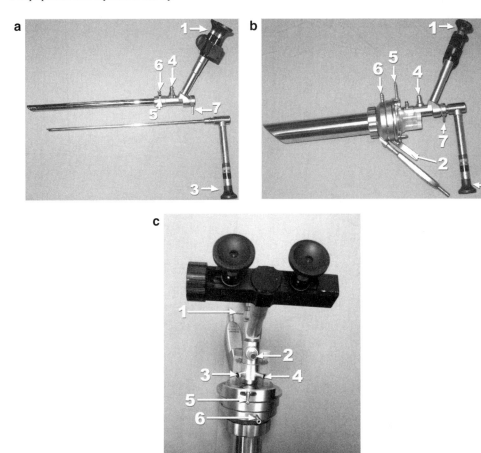

Fig. 3.5 a Optic system. *1* binocular eye pieces, *3* the attachment site for the monocular optic to the video monitor, *4* light cord attachment, *5* CO_2 insufflation tube port, *6* water-infusion port, *7* lock for monocular optic. **b** *1* binocular eye pieces, *2* lock for faceplate, *3* video attachment to monocular optic, *4* light cord attachment, *5* lock for binocular scope, *6* port for CO_2 pressure monitor tube, *7* lock for monocular optic. **c** Closeup of operating proctoscope. *1* lock for monocular optic, *2* light cord attachment, *3* port for CO_2 insufflation, *4* port for water infusion, *5* lock for binocular optic, *6* port for CO_2 pressure monitor tube

pedal. The pistol grip, utilizing the ulnar grip portion of the hand, is ergonometrically designed for operations that require holding the knife for prolonged periods.

The long forceps have two types of tips, either straight or angled. Both types are provided on instruments with tips facing towards either the left or the right. Each instrument may be electrified; they are insulated, and have a fitting for attachment of an electrocautery cord. The jaws of the forceps are designed for holding tissue at the tip, but further back the jaws are ridged for gripping and receiving a suture needle being passed through tissue. The scissors are provided with the tip facing either left or right, and are mainly used for cutting sutures.

The suction probe is a long, double-curved, rigid tube that is designed to be inserted through the proctoscope and sit to the side of the scope away from the center of the

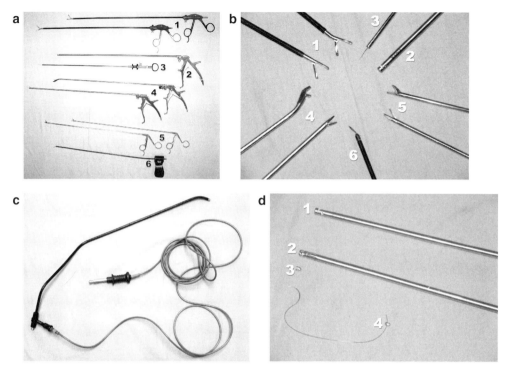

Fig. 3.6 a Long operating instruments. *1* forceps with tip angles, left and right, *2* clip applier, *3* retractable injection needle, *4* needle holders, both angled and straight tip, *5* scissors angled both right and left, *6* electric knife. **b** Long operating instrument tips. *1* forceps angled right and left, *2* clip applier, *3* retractable injection needle, *4* needle holders with angled and straight tips, *5* electric knife. *6* scissors angled right and left. **c** Suction probe. Note that it is double-angled to keep the probe out of the way of straight operating instruments. The probe can be electrified with the cord attached. **d** Clip appliers. *1* tip of empty clip applier, *2* clip applier loaded with silver clip, *3* silver clip, *4* clip crimped onto suture tip

operative field (Fig. 3.6c). The suction is generally placed through the lower, center operating port, and can be used by the surgeon or an assistant to remove blood, liquid stool, and smoke. There is a connection for attaching the electrocautery. It is insulated except for the suction/cautery tip permitting electrocoagulation, but preventing accidental coagulation away from the tip. Thus, blood can be suctioned while coagulating a bleeding vessel.

The needle device has a retractable needle within the tip of the rigid tube and may be extended or retracted with the syringe type handle. There is a Luer lock on the side of the device for the injection of solutions, such as a dilute epinephrine for hemostasis or India ink for tattooing.

The needle holders are available with either a straight or an angled tip (Fig. 3.6b). The angled tip provides a slightly wider arc when the surgeon is passing a needle. In addition the jaws are "self-righting" so when the needle is grasped it will rotate into the proper orientation. The needle can be locked in position with a rotating ratchet controlled by the surgeon's thumb. The lock is released by oversqueezing the handle, allowing the surgeon to safely manipulate the needle.

The clip applier is a unique instrument (Fig. 3.6d) which crimps a small silver clip onto the suture. Clips are placed at the beginning and the end of running suture, replacing the

3 Equipment and Operative Set-up

need for knot tying. The operating room technician places a silver clip on the suture at 6–7 cm from the needle in preparation for suturing. A second clip is placed on the suture by the surgeon to complete a running suture line.

Insufflator/Suction/Irrigation/Light/Electrocautery Machines

The video monitor and machines for CO_2 insufflation, water injection, light, and suction are stacked on a portable cart (Fig. 3.7). An electrocoagulation machine may be placed in the stack of machines on the cart or a standard operating room machine may be employed. The insufflator introduces CO_2 via a port on the binocular optic shaft. Light is delivered via a fiberoptic cord to a connection on the binocular optic probe (Fig. 3.5b). Water may be switched on using a pedal. Water is driven by CO_2 pressure which is delivered to a water reservoir and which is, in turn, driven to the port on the stereoscope shaft. The water travels through the stereoscope shaft and is directed across the optic at the tip for cleaning and irrigation. The pedal may be tapped (for less than 0.5 s), and the suction roller pump will work maximally. Tap again and the roller pump will return to the preset rate. Hold the

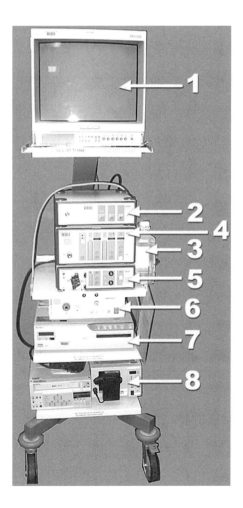

Fig. 3.7 Transanal endoscopic microsurgery (TEM) cart. *1* monitor, *2* camera, *3* irrigation reservoir, *4* Insufflator, *5* TEM pump, *6* light source, *7* Printer, *8* Digital Video Disk Recorder

pedal down, and it will irrigate for 4s. Repeated pressing causes continuous flow of whatever volume of water is desired.

Adaptable Laparoscopic Instruments

Harmonic Scalpel

A special harmonic scalpel has been designed for laparoscopic surgery (Fig. 3.8). It is a high-energy ultrasonic vibrator (55,500 cycles/s), which mechanically denatures tissue proteins, resulting in cavitation and sealing of blood vessels. The ultrasonic shears have a blunt vibrating blade and a narrow closure blade. The shears coagulate most vessels up to 5-mm diameter with minimal vapor production. However, the instrument tip does become hot enough to burn adjacent tissues if touched.

LigaSure

LigaSure is a vessel-sealing device which delivers electrical energy through special graspers (Fig. 3.9). A high coaptive pressure with a temperature greater than 100°C denatures

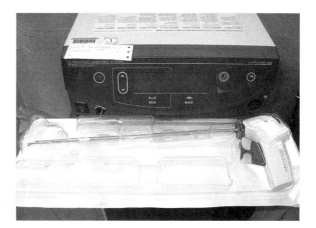

Fig. 3.8 Harmonic scalpel power box and disposable shears

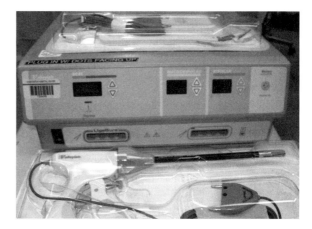

Fig. 3.9 LigaSure vessel-sealing device and disposable graspers

3 Equipment and Operative Set-up   21

collagen and elastin, permanently sealing blood vessel walls. The device has a pistol grip, and a trigger-operated blade to cut and separate the sealed vessel ends.

Surgical Set-up

Assembling the equipment can be time-consuming, and if there is a failure in the system, troubleshooting can result in significant delays. The team, consisting of the surgeon, assistant, scrub nurse, and circulating nurse, have different responsibilities in setting up for a TEM procedure.

The surgeon must position the patient with the tumor directly down toward the operating table; the choice of position is based upon the examination in the office with a rigid proctoscope locating the tumor at both a specific level and a specific site on the circumference. The patient may be placed in the lithotomy position, prone, or laterally; for a tumor that is circumferential the patient may need to be turned during the procedure. The patient must be secured to the table by straps, tape, and perhaps with a bean bag, as the table may need to be rotated to bring the tumor into the center of the field. For the lateral position, a clamp-on table must be attached to the bottom of the operating table to support the legs extended at right angles, allowing the perineum to reach the bottom of the operating table (alternatively split leg attachments can be used) (Fig 3.10a). The lithotomy position may be maintained with rigid or candy cane stirrups. The most difficult position is prone, which requires the legs be in jackknife angulation. The knees can be supported on a shelf that is

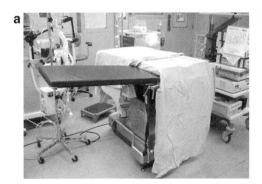
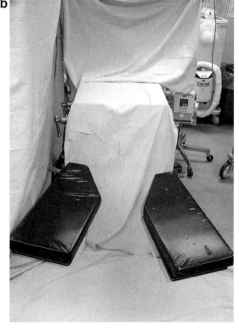

Fig. 3.10 a Operating table with attached table to support the legs in lateral position. **b** Operating table with attached adjustable leg supports for the prone position

usually standard equipment with the operating table unit, or special leg supports that can be individually rotated may be purchased for this specific indication (Fig. 3.10b).

After draping, the articulated arm is attached via a clamp to one of the rails on the operating table. The four tubes leaving the insufflation/suction apparatus and cords must be properly connected.

The scrub nurse checks to see that the handles and jaws of the instruments function correctly. The washers to prevent gas leak on the faceplates are attached. The tips of the stereoscopes and monocular scopes are warmed in water and antifog solution is applied to the optics. Long-acting local anesthetic with epinephrine is made available for an anal block and injection around the tumor site for hemostasis. The sutures are made ready with a silver clip applied 6–7 cm from the needle. (Fig. 3.6b) Generally 3-O polydioxanone is used as the suture. A cap is back-loaded on the needle holder, which is later pushed onto the operating port to maintain an airtight seal. Water-soluble lubricant is applied near the tip of all instruments to minimize friction while sliding through the cap.

The circulating nurse must be educated in setting up and starting the machines that serve the TEM system. The power sources are connected. The CO_2 tank must have adequate volume. The TEM cart with the monitor is placed to the right side of the operating table in view of the surgeon, assistant, and scrub nurse. If video documentation is planned, a videotape or DVD is inserted. After the patient enters the room, the identification and allergies are checked. A urinary catheter and compression stockings are applied. The surgeon will often need to help with positioning to match the known position of the tumor in the rectum. Pressure points are padded and a grounding pad is applied.

The sterile light source and electrocautery cords are attached to the field and the ends are passed off to the circulating nurse; then the machines are turned on; the pedal for the electrocautery is placed near the surgeon's foot. The irrigation pedal is attached to the electrical connecting post on the back of the machine, and is placed where it can be reached easily by the surgeon.

The steps in starting the insufflation machine must be performed in an exact order, otherwise the whole process must be stopped and (after waiting 30s) restarted. These ordered steps bear listing so that they will be performed correctly at each use:

1. The on/off switch is pressed (Fig. 3.11a) An alternating yellow/green flashing light signal goes on (Fig. 3.11a), indicating that the machine is undergoing diagnostic tests and is self-calibrating. When the signal light becomes a steady green, the process may proceed.
2. The roller pump tubing is placed into the roller pump; the round side of the gray tab is inserted into the upper slot; the tube is manually rotated around the roller; then the round end of the red tab is pushed into the red slot (Fig. 3.11a)
3. The nonfilter end of the short irrigation pressure tube is attached to the irrigation bottle, and the filter end is attached to the insufflation machine (Fig. 3.11b). This tube delivers CO_2 into the bottle to create the pressure that will drive the water through the stereoscope.
4. The sterile four tube combination set is fixed to the operating field, and the ends with the CO_2 filter are passed to the circulating nurse for attachment to the insufflation machine. The large CO_2 filter is connected to the large port (Fig. 3.11b). The red-tipped tube is attached to the suction tube exiting the roller pump. The remaining free end of the tubing exiting the roller pump is placed in a receptacle to receive fluid suctioned from the operative field. The blue-tipped tubing is connected to the water bottle (Fig. 3.11b). The rectal pressure monitoring tube with the green filter is attached (Fig. 3.11b).

3 Equipment and Operative Set-up

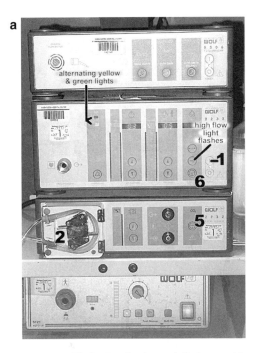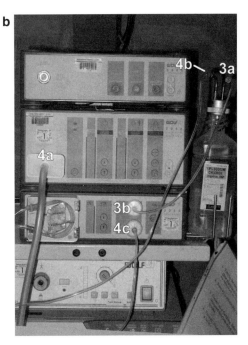

Fig. 3.11 Insufflation/suction/water-infusion machine; steps for turning the unit on. The numbered steps are consecutive in **a** and **b**. **a** *1* press the on/off power button—alternating green and yellow lights as the machine self-calibrates and self-tests, *2* the suction tubing is placed on the roller pump, *5* the TEM mode button is pushed—the high-flow light flashes; *6* the gas-flow button is pushed. **b** *3a* attachment of gas-insufflation tube to water reservoir, *3b* attachment of gas filter to water line, *4a* attachment of CO_2 line filter, *4b* attachment of the water line to the reservoir, *4c* attachment of the filter from the CO_2 pressure monitor line

5. The on/off switch of the TEM pump is turned to on and (Fig. 3.11a) the high-flow button flashes, showing that the TEM mode is on.
6. The primary insufflation flow button can now be pushed (Fig. 3.11a).
7. The front of the machine has several LCD display bars (Fig. 3.12) which indicate the maximum CO_2 flow rate and the actual flow rate. In addition, another display identifies intrarectal pressure, both maximum and current pressure.

Troubleshooting

Technical failures will occur and require a systematic approach to trouble shooting. A series of problems will be presented with appropriate solutions.

Prior to the operation, the machine does not work. Check to see if there is power in the outlet and that the power cable is connected. A faulty fuse may be the cause and if so an indicator on the insufflator will read "ERR."

The pneumorectum is not adequate or is leaking. The CO_2 tank may be empty or low. One of the locks or caps is loose. The insufflation tubing may be kinked or loose at one of the ends. The CO_2 flow rate may be set too low. Some instruments have hollow shafts with Luer lock type connections which must be capped. Finally, there may be a leak around the

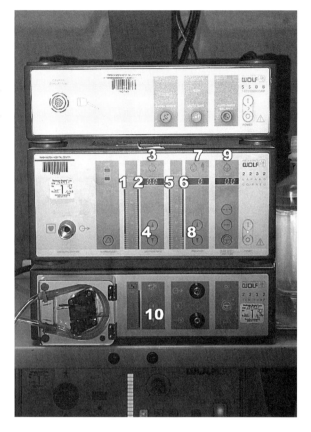

Fig. 3.12 Gauges and regulating buttons. *1* preset vertical gas flow bar, *2* actual gas flow bar, *3* digital reading of gas flow, *4* buttons for increasing and decreasing gas flow, *5* preset vertical gas pressure bar, *6* actual gas pressure bar, *7* digital reading of gas pressure, *8* buttons for regulation of gas pressure, *9* digital reading of gas volume used, *10* buttons for regulation of suction roller pump rate

proctoscope at the anal level; this is particularly true when working at a low level in the rectum. The rectal pressure measuring line is on the rear of the machine, which could be ajar and leaking, a hidden site to check.

If the lighting is a problem, the problem usually occurs at the start of the procedure. Increase the gain and see that the light comes through the cable. A light may indicate the machine is in standby mode. A loose connection can be quickly adjusted. If the fiberoptic cord is damaged, it must be replaced. If there is no light, the bulb may need to be replaced. If the image is dark, recheck the white balance. Turning down the room lights improves the image as well.

A picture on the monitor may be flickering or of poor quality. The camera head, cables, and white balance may be at fault. If there is no picture, all cables and power sources should be checked. Poor quality of the picture may be due to fogging. Detach the camera and clean the lens as necessary. The tip may simply need to be warmed and antifog solution applied. A blurred image is often corrected by adjusting the focus ring. If a lens is cracked permitting moisture to enter the camera, it must be exchanged.

Inadequate suction or irrigation is often due to kinking or clogging; inspection will find the site quickly. The tubes pressuring the fluid container may be ajar and may be reconnected. All connections can be checked and adjusted. Adjust suction settings as necessary.

Electrocautery may be weak or absent. Individual machines have their own problems, but some are universal. Check the grounding pad and connections. The foot pedal may not be connected. A cable may not be plugged into the correct socket on the machine or the instrument.

Occasionally communication with the equipment service representatives or the biomedical engineers at your hospital may be necessary.

Conclusions

TEM requires specialized equipment and training. In addition to technical expertise, the dedicated TEM surgeon should be familiar with the necessary instruments and electronic devices. Expertise in troubleshooting is particularly helpful. There is, however, no substitute for a dedicated operating room team consisting of a circulating nurse, technician, and available biomedical engineer to facilitate smooth, efficient, successful TEM.

Chapter 4
Pelvic Anatomic Considerations for Transanal Endoscopic Microsurgery

Peter A. Cataldo

The rectum is a complex structure, protected from harm by multiple anatomic guardians. These structures not only protect the rectum from external trauma, but also make surgical access exceptionally difficult. This complex organ, essential for socially acceptable elimination of intestinal waste, is most obviously protected by the bony pelvis, but also by the anal sphincters below and by the abdominal contents above.

These protective structures, which limit surgical access to the rectum, are responsible for the development of transanal endoscopic microsurgery (TEM). If access to the rectum were unlimited, there would be no need for TEM. The inability of transanal, transsphincteric, transcoccygeal, and transabdominal approaches to provide safe, reliable exposure to allow for local excision of rectal masses is the stimulus that led to the creation of TEM in 1983. A long operating proctoscope, superior optics, specialized instrumentation, and rectal insufflation together have overcome the obstacles of the formidable pelvic structures and allow for safe consistent excision of masses throughout the rectum.

Even with the advent of TEM, the vagaries of pelvic anatomy still create problems limiting the surgeon's ability to remove certain rectal masses. In addition, the crowded nature of the pelvic anatomy and the essential structures in immediate proximity lead to specific complications, not necessarily limited to, but certainly closely associated with TEM.

Rectal Access

The access needed for TEM is by definition via the anal orifice. This first barrier is almost always traversable, but not without cost. In rare cases of anal stenosis, secondary to prior anal surgery (such as radical hemorrhoidectomy) or significant excision of anal canal skin for squamous cell cancer, Bowen's disease, or anal condyloma access may be impossible; but these are truly rare exceptions.

Even if proctoscopic insertion is uneventful, it may not be without consequence. Advancing a 40-mm TEM scope through all but the most patulous anus requires substantial anal dilatation. Both the internal and the external anal sphincters are affected. Kreis et al. [1] found consistent decreases in resting anal tone and squeeze pressure following TEM. Hermann et al. [2] identified sphincteric defects by endoscopic ultrasound in 29% of patients undergoing TEM. Kennedy et al. [3] found increasing length of procedure

---

P.A. Cataldo (✉)
University of Vermont College of Medicine, Burlington, VT, USA

P.A. Cataldo, G.F. Buess (eds.), *Transanal Endoscopic Microsurgery*,
DOI 10.1007/978-0-387-76397-2_4, © Springer Science+Business Media, LLC 2009

associated with decreased internal sphincter function postoperatively. Also, large-volume rectal resections and preoperative impairment of continence were associated with compromised postoperative function [2, 3]. However, Cataldo et al. [4], in the largest study comparing preoperative and postoperative continence, found no change in defecatory function following TEM for both benign and malignant rectal masses. In summary, the anal sphincters provide the "protective gate" that must be transversed in order to perform TEM, but in most patients this can be accomplished without significant anatomic or functional consequences.

The Rectum

The rectum appears in most textbooks to be essentially straight and easily traversable; however, anyone who routinely performs, or has personally experienced, rigid sigmoidoscopy knows differently (Fig. 4.1). Any difficulty accessing the rectum with a 10-mm sigmoidoscope is magnified substantially when using a 40-mm TEM proctoscope. There are several locations within the rectum that are particularly challenging to expose with TEM. The first is the very distal rectum just above the anorectal junction. At the very distal limits of the rectum, short anal canal length can lead to difficulty "maintaining a seal" around the proctoscope, with secondary incomplete pneumorectum and poor visualization. This is particularly problematic when trying to close a defect created by excising a low rectal mass. The excision will often proceed without incident, but the additional distal exposure necessary for wound closure may be very difficult. In this circumstance, it is often better to remove the TEM proctoscope and close the defect via a standard transanal approach. For large lesions, if the proximal rectal resection line is out of reach, placing one or two traction sutures proximally prior to removing the TEM proctoscope will allow the surgeon to pull the upper rectal resection line distally to facilitate closure.

The second anatomic challenge lies posteriorly just proximal to the anorectal junction. Above the puborectalis, in some individuals, the rectal ampulla extends sharply and abruptly posteriorly (Fig. 4.2). Lesions just above the anorectal junction may be very difficult to "center" in the TEM field owing to the inflexibility of the proctoscope and the sharp angulation of the anorectal junction. In this circumstance, proper positioning is very helpful. The patient's legs should be in a very high lithotomy position and the operating room table in a significant reverse Trendelenburg position. These two maneuvers will minimize the anorectal angle and allow the proctoscope to be directed at distal posterior rectal lesions.

The next rectal obstacles are the valves of Houston. These are the prominent folds that exist in the distal, middle, and proximal rectum. Occasionally, a sessile polyp may lie on the proximal or "top side" of these folds, making complete exposure challenging. In this case it is occasionally necessary to partially excise the valve in order to completely visualize and excise the lesion.

The final extrinsic rectal anatomic detail affecting TEM is the curvature at the rectosigmoid junction. Many times, particularly in patients having prior abdominal or pelvic surgery, there is a very sharp angulation at this junction. The ability to pass a rigid sigmoidoscope in the office at the time of preoperative evaluation is usually predictive of successful TEM exposure. However, in some circumstances the large diameter of the operating proctoscope may prohibit exposure at the time of TEM. While advancing the proctoscope completely separating it from the Martin arm may facilitate proximal exposure, forceful advancement of the scope can lead to full-thickness tears in the rectal

4 Pelvic Anatomic Considerations for Transanal Endoscopic Microsurgery

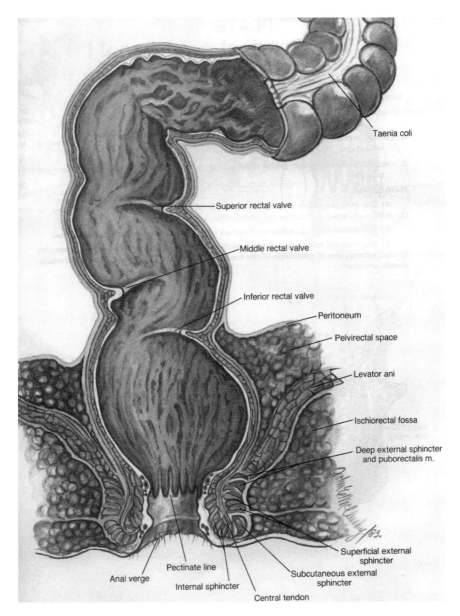

Fig. 4.1 The rectum appears relatively straight in most anatomic drawings, but the anorectal junction, the valves of Houston, and the rectosigmoid junction can be significant barriers to passage of the proctoscope. (Gray SW, Skandalakis JE, McClusky DA. Atlas of Surgical Anatomy for General Surgeons. Williams & Wilkins, 1985.)

wall particularly adjacent to the sacrum. In this situation, it is better to abandon TEM in favor of a transabdominal approach.

In addition to the natural rectal obstacles, "man-made" obstacles also exist, and these may create a more substantial challenge. Luminal stenosis, most commonly the result of multiple attempts at endoscopic excision of a large rectal polyp or due to a large rectal tumor, may prevent proximal passage of the proctoscope, leading to inadequate exposure.

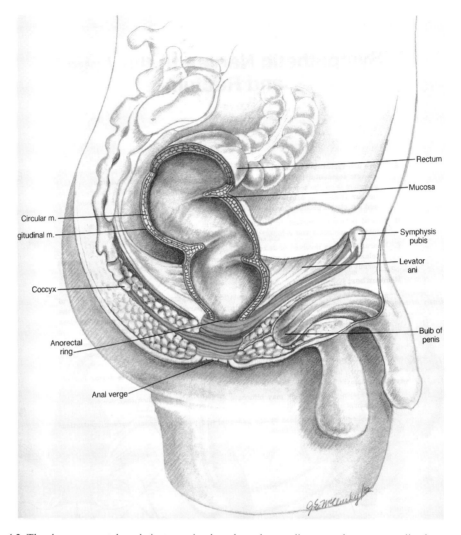

Fig. 4.2 The sharp anorectal angle just proximal to the puborectalis can make access to distal, posterior rectal masses difficult. (Gray SW, Skandalakis JE, McClusky DA. Atlas of Surgical Anatomy for General Surgeons. Williams & Wilkins, 1985.)

In these cases, it is often necessary to begin the dissection and excision distal to the level of the stenosis and to proceed proximally in the extrarectal plane until the lesion has been removed.

Extrarectal Anatomy

While intrinsic anal and rectal anatomies predict accessibility and resectability, it is extrarectal anatomy that predicts complications (Fig. 4.3). The mesorectum lies predominantly posterior to the rectum and has gained worldwide importance in transabdominal rectal excision. This is due to the fact that the blood supply to the rectum arises through the mesorectum, and perhaps more importantly, the lymphatic and the venous drainage exit the rectum here. In performing TEM, the mesorectum is important for two reasons. Firstly,

4 Pelvic Anatomic Considerations for Transanal Endoscopic Microsurgery

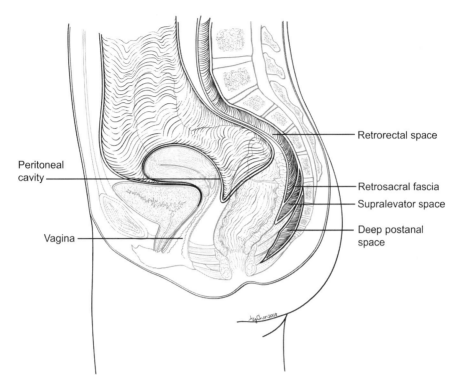

Fig. 4.3 The mesorectum lies directly posterior to the rectum, and the prostate and vagina directly anterior. All are at risk during transanal endoscopic microsurgery. (Adapted from Fig. 12 of Gordon and Nivatvongs [6] with permission from Informa Healthcare)

large blood vessels may penetrate the posterior rectal wall, leading to excessive bleeding if not carefully controlled. Judicious use of electrocautery, or alternatively the Harmonic Scalpel or LigaSure may be very beneficial. Secondly, generous excision of the mesorectum when performing TEM for malignancy may yield one or more lymph nodes, which in some cases alters preoperative staging. Sentinal node technology has been applied to the mesorectum and has been successful at identifying lymph nodes. Unfortunately, these nodes have not been predictive of other mesorectal adenopathy. Currently, several new technologies are being applied in this area to help identify metastatic lymph nodes in patients undergoing local excision of rectal cancer.

Most significant anatomic structures lie anterior to the rectum and these are particularly at risk during TEM. In men, only a thin layer of Denonvillier's fascia separates the rectum from the prostate. Fortunately, injury to the prostatic urethra is exceptionally rare: however, significant bleeding can result from prostatic veins if dissection extends too far anteriorly in the distal rectum.

In women, the anovaginal septum resides immediately anterior to the distal third of the rectum, beginning at the level of the anal canal. This anatomic barrier is variable in thickness and can be virtually nonexistent in women who have had significant anal sphincter disruptions as a result of vaginal delivery or in women with large rectoceles. In these circumstances, it is very easy to enter the posterior vagina while dissecting the deep plane in full-thickness excisions of anterior rectal masses. This is usually recognized immediately as the rectum rapidly collapses owing to the loss of CO_2 through the vaginal defect. The defect can be closed via TEM or via a traditional approach after removing the TEM equipment. Failure to recognize this injury universally leads to a postoperative rectovaginal fistula.

Peritoneal Reflections

The rectum sits in the true pelvis and is tangentially divided in half by the pelvic peritoneum (Fig. 4.4). The relationship between the peritoneum and the rectum is possibly the most important aspect of pelvic anatomy that pertains to TEM. Techniques useful in the extraperitoneal rectum, such as leaving rectal defects open to close by secondary intention, result in disastrous complications (peritonitis) if employed in the intraperitoneal rectum. In addition, full-thickness excision of rectal malignancy in the intraperitoneal portions of the rectum may potentially lead to dissemination of aerosolized tumor cells into the peritoneal cavity. This theoretically can result in tumor implantation and subsequent pelvic, peritoneal metastases (which the author has seen on one occasion).

The peritoneum transverses the rectum from cephalad to caudad in a posterior to anterior fashion; thus, the entire posterior rectum is extraperitoneal, while the lateral aspects of the rectum are extraperitoneal in the distal two thirds, and the anterior rectum is extraperitoneal only in the distal one third. This relationship varies among individuals. Women with rectal prolapse have a very deep anterior peritoneal reflection and therefore

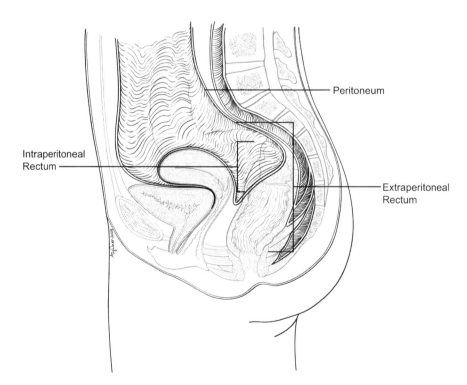

Fig. 4.4 Peritoneal reflections The peritoneum transverses the rectum from posterior to anterior in a cephalad to caudad direction leaving large portions of the anterior rectum intraperitoneal. (Adapted from Fig. 4 of Gordon and Nivatvongs [6] with permission from Informa Healthcare)

their entire anterior rectum may be intraperitoneal. Men may have a high peritoneal reflection, leaving the majority of their anterior rectum intraperitoneal. However, a study performed by Najarian et al. [5] indicated the mean distance of the anterior peritoneal reflections to be very similar in men and women, 9.7 and 9.0 cm, respectively. Another important factor often unappreciated is the "thickness" of the peritoneal envelope. Posterior rectal locations just above the anorectal junction have a large extrarectal space with a significant barrier to the intraperitoneal cavity. Conversely, as one gets closer to the intraperitoneal rectum the "peritoneal barrier" becomes very thin and cannot be safely relied upon to prevent intraperitoneal spread of fecal contents.

After extensive experience with full-thickness TEM resections of the rectum, one finds the peritoneal reflections to be very variable in their location and thickness. Except in very unusual circumstances, therefore, primary closure of all rectal defects is prudent. This minimizes any worry about intraperitoneal fecal contamination and may also minimize postoperative bleeding. In addition, although not clearly supported in the literature, primary closure of extraperitoneal rectal defects may facilitate postoperative recovery. Finally, and perhaps most importantly, routine closure of all rectal defects hones the surgeon's TEM suturing techniques, allowing for secure, comfortable closure when intraperitoneal rectal resections are necessary or encountered unexpectedly.

Conclusions

TEM facilitates access throughout the entire rectum, allowing surgeons to resect lesions previously inaccessible by traditional techniques. With this additional access comes increased opportunity for complications; these complications are very dependent upon anatomic relationships between the rectum and the surrounding structures. As in any surgical procedure, intricate knowledge and comprehensive understanding of this complex pelvic anatomy will significantly minimize the risk of anatomic, postoperative complications.

References

1. Kreis ME, Jehle EC, Haug V, et al. Functional results after transanal endoscopic microsurgery. *Dis Colon Rectum* 1996;39:1116–21.
2. Herman RM, Richter P, Walega P, et al. Anorectal sphincter function and rectal barostat study in patients following transanal endoscopic microsurgery. *Int J Colorectal Dis* 2001;6:370–6.
3. Kennedy ML, Lubowski DZ, King DW, et al. Transanal endoscopic microsurgery excision: is anorectal function compromised? *Dis Colon Rectum* 2002;45:601–4.
4. Cataldo PA, O'Brien S, Osler T. Transanal endoscopic microsurgery: a prospective evaluation of functional results *Dis Colon Rectum* 2004;481366–1371.
5. Najarian MM, Belzer GE, Cogbill TH, Mathiason MA. Determination of the peritoneal reflection using intraoperative proctoscopy. *Dis Colon Rectum* 2004 47(12):2080–2085.
6. Gordon PH, Nivatvongs S. Principles and practices of surgery of colon, rectum, and anus, 3rd edn, 2007, Informa Healthcare, New York.

Chapter 5
Getting Started

Patricia L. Roberts

Transanal endoscopic microsurgery (TEM) was developed by Buess in 1983 and involves the use of specialized equipment to remove selected rectal cancers and polyps [1]. The equipment involves an operating proctoscope, insufflation, and magnified stereoscopic vision to improve visualization and facilitate more precise excision. Although there are approximately 430 TEM systems in use worldwide, there are only approximately 45 active units in the USA. Adoption of the technique of TEM has been slow in the USA probably because of the cost of the unit and the challenges of adequate training [2]. Despite these challenges, the improved visualization and optics of TEM combined with the ability to remove lesions throughout the rectum appear to have ensured the role of TEM in the surgeon's armamentarium. This chapter reviews the steps in beginning a TEM program, including the decision to pursue TEM equipment, training, the early experience, and the learning curve.

Deciding To Pursue Transanal Endoscopic Microsurgery

TEM expands the armamentarium of the surgeon for local excision of selected rectal cancers and polyps. While benign rectal polyps of the distal rectum can be excised by standard transanal approaches, selected polyps of the mid rectum or more proximal rectum may be uniquely suited to the performance of TEM. These lesions traditionally have been treated by an abdominal procedure such as low anterior resection.

Although polyps and selected cancers may be treated by TEM, the numbers of cases in any one surgical practice is generally not very large, and therefore it is prudent for one or two members of a group, not the entire group, to be trained in the technique. If all members of the group attempt to dabble in the technique, it is unlikely any one individual will be able to develop sufficient expertise. Conversely, it is advisable for a core group of operating room nurses to gain proficiency in the setup and use of the equipment.

Purchasing the equipment and gaining expertise with the technique does not necessarily increase the number of cases of transanal excision at an institution [2]. Some institutions have found that the availability of the equipment has increased referrals for rectal cancers but has not impacted on the percentage of lesions amenable to local excision. Of all rectal cancers, generally fewer than 10% are amenable to local excision [3, 4]. Therefore, it is

---

P.L. Roberts (✉)
Tufts University School of Medicine, Boston, MA, Lahey Clinic, Burlington, MA, USA

P.A. Cataldo, G.F. Buess (eds.), *Transanal Endoscopic Microsurgery*,
DOI 10.1007/978-0-387-76397-2_5, © Springer Science+Business Media, LLC 2009

essential that an individual or institution has a sufficient volume of rectal abnormalities amenable to TEM prior to developing a program in TEM.

Equipment Available

TEM equipment was first developed by Wolf Surgical Instruments (Vernon Hills, IL, USA) and is also currently available through Karl Storz (Tuttlingen, Germany). The instruments are prepackaged as a set containing all necessary equipment to perform TEM. A trainer set is also available to practice the procedure in a skills laboratory setting. Bovine large intestine, which is available for purchase through slaughterhouses, is the best material for training; however, as many institutions prohibit use of instruments on animals if they are then to be used in humans, use of bovine bowel may be prohibited, in which case an inanimate trainer can be used.

The TEM equipment is held in place by a Martin arm, a multielbowed holder which is attached to the operating room table. The proctoscope can then be placed precisely and locked into position. Operating proctoscopes are available in different lengths, but all are 4 cm in diameter. Gentle rectal dilatation is necessary before placing the proctoscope. The scope is then placed with the beveled end downward. It is essential to position the patient so that the lesion is in the "bottom half" of the field; therefore, patients with posteriorly located lesions should be placed in the lithotomy position, and patients with anteriorly located lesions should be placed in the prone position. Split-leg table attachments are useful. For lateral lesions, patients are placed in the appropriate lateral decubitus position. Once the lesion has been visualized, the removable faceplate, which has four ports, is attached and locked into place. One port is for the optical stereoscope, one is for suction, and the other two are for placement of instruments to perform TEM. Conduits for insufflation, irrigation, a light cord, and a pressure transducer are attached to the stereoscope and faceplate. The stereoscope is a 10-mm instrument with a 50° downward viewing angle and two eyepieces for viewing. An additional 40° 5-mm scope is attached and thus the procedure can also be viewed on a standard laparoscopic monitor.

TEM uses a closed endoscopic system that provides for simultaneous CO_2 insufflation and measurement of intrarectal pressure, which is usually set at a desired level of 10–15 cm H_2O. It is essential for the system to be airtight. Once the faceplate has been attached, the TEM tubing is attached. This must be accomplished in the proper sequence or the unit will not function properly. There are four pieces of tubing, including one for insufflation, one for continuous monitoring of intrarectal pressure, another for irrigation of the lens and the operative field, and a fourth for roller-pump suction. Roller-pump suction must be used since conventional suction will instantly deflate the entire rectal lumen.

Once setup has been accomplished, excision of the lesion can be performed. A local anesthetic solution with epinephrine is injected and the appropriate margin then marked with the electrocautery. A submucosal or full-thickness excision can be carried out depending on whether the lesion is benign or malignant, respectively. From a technical standpoint, a full-thickness excision is easier and the presence of the yellow perirectal fat is the hallmark of the appropriate plane. In general, the lesion is excised from distal to proximal, and for the right-handed surgeon, from right to left. While the electrocautery is generally used for excision, some groups have suggested that the harmonic scalpel is associated with less smoke and better visualization [5]. During the dissection, it is helpful to assess the margins of resection for time to time; one of the pitfalls is dissecting too far proximally and undermining the lesion.

Once the lesion has been removed, it is retrieved by opening the faceplate. Small defects, particularly posterior defects which are extraperitoneal, may be left open. It has been suggested that closing the defects improves skills and should be performed since it is easy to have a small unrecognized intraperitoneal perforation [6]. Suturing the defect is more difficult than actually performing the excision. This can be done in several ways. For intraluminal suturing (the most difficult), a metal bead (silver bb) is attached at the beginning with the use of a crimper and the defect is closed with a running stitch with a bb on the end. Care is taken to ensure that the lumen is not compromised and proctoscopy is performed at the conclusion of the procedure to ensure that the lumen is patent. Some groups have found that use of an extracorporeal slip knot facilitates closure and have termed this a "hybrid approach" as it uses TEM and traditional transanal techniques [5]. We have, on many occasions, found it easier to removed the faceplate and perform conventional suturing utilizing the laparoscopic clip applier to secure the stitch on either end.

Training the Team

Once the decision has been made to acquire TEM equipment and to start the program, the team members must be trained. This includes both the surgeon and the operating room staff (generally scrub and circulating nurses and surgical technicians).

Prior to beginning the program, a didactic course with hands-on training is essential. Courses are generally given several times a year and are available at national meetings (including those of the American Society of Colon and Rectal Surgeons and the Society of Gastrointestinal Endoscopic Surgeons). The surgeon must concentrate both on proficiency with the use of the equipment (particularly equipment setup and troubleshooting) and on proficiency with the technique. Optimally, the team should train together, particularly with respect to troubleshooting and equipment setup. We have found it helpful to have a nurse train at a facility that has a high volume of TEM procedures. Following this training, several "dry runs" can be performed to set up the unit. A laminated card with the bulleted points for setup is placed on the unit to assist in troubleshooting. Alternatively, if a course is not available, separate arrangements can be made for the surgeon to train with another surgeon who performs a large number of TEM procedures.

There are several important points for the beginning TEM surgeon to recognize. The tendency is to think of the technique as being similar to laparoscopic surgery; while there are common elements, such as working off a monitor, there are important differences. The instruments must be used in a single up-and-down axis which has been likened to a piston. Crossover of the instruments in the confined space used to perform TEM is not possible. The instruments used to perform TEM must be used in parallel, in contrast to the preferred 90° orientation in laparoscopy. There is little ability to use an assistant, and therefore the surgeon must be able to provide his or her own "traction/countertraction" of the lesion to facilitate the dissection. While in laparoscopic surgery, another port site can be inserted to assist, this is not possible in TEM [7].

Care should be taken to position the patient appropriately. For ease of performance of the procedure, it is essential to have the lesion in the lower portion of the operating field. Thus, for posterior lesions, the patient is placed in the lithotomy position, for anterior lesions in the prone position, and for right lateral and left lateral lesions in the right and left lateral decubitus positions, respectively.

The surgeon should be able to troubleshoot since seemingly "minor" problems may preclude proper functioning of the equipment. One common issue is collapse of the operative field; if this occurs, the procedure cannot be performed. This problem can occur from cracks in the rubber caps or sleeves, failure to lock the faceplate or scope in place, or kinking of the CO_2 gas line.

Initially, additional time should be set aside to perform a TEM procedure. With increased experience, operative times decrease [8]. Some groups have found that operative time has had an impact on continence [9], while others have not [10]. The impact on minor changes in continence is presumably from the dilatation of the anal canal necessary to insert the operating proctoscope.

Following training at a course, it is important to be able to continually use the newly acquired skills. Ongoing or weekly training sessions are valuable in a skills laboratory setting. Owing to the cost of the equipment, most centers do not have an extra set of equipment for use in the skills laboratory with animal parts, and thus achieving proficiency and maintaining skills is difficult. Human intestine can be used for basic suturing and to practice resection, but we have found it inadequate for maintaining insufflation and therefore inadequate for performing all facets of the procedure. Others have suggested that practicing using the equipment through a cardboard tube, such as a paper towel roll, can assist with avoiding instrument crossover and working in parallel.

Early Experience and Patient Selection

We have found the following points to be helpful in the early experience of TEM. These points are not meant to be prescriptive, but to represent potential helpful hints.

The initial lesions selected for a TEM procedure should be lesions amenable to conventional techniques of transanal excision. A small mobile and easily visualized lesion is optimal. While it is suggested that lesions up to 25 cm may be amenable to TEM, lesions in the distal to mid rectum are easier to tackle in the early experience. If a lesion is too close to the anal verge however, maintaining insufflation will be challenging owing to difficulty maintaining an airtight seal in the distal anal canal. In addition, proximity to the hemorrhoid columns can be associated with increased bleeding and subsequent difficulty with visualization. In our early experience, we have removed several 1-cm carcinoid tumors and small residual polyps which, owing to their sessile and/or submucosal nature, could not be removed endoscopically. The lesions selected in the initial experience should be well within the extraperitoneal rectum. While intraperitoneal lesions can be removed by "expert" and experienced TEM surgeons, these lesions are not advisable in the early experience. Entry into the peritoneum is challenging to manage and must be closed securely. In addition, other groups have found that higher lesions are associated with a higher rate of conversion to another procedure, such as low anterior resection [11]. In one series of 144 consecutive TEM procedures, the position of the lesion was evaluated by spatial analysis using geographic information systems and then related to the ability to perform the procedure. Conversions were more likely in more proximal lesion ($P < 0.05$) [11]. In addition, with posterior lesions, patient positioning is simple, while anterior lesions can be challenging, even with a split table.

Case Booking

We have found it optimal to schedule the procedure for the first operation of the day. In our experience, the trained nurses are available then and are less likely to be pulled for another procedure. Allocate extra time to ensure adequate setup and patient positioning.

Case Setup and Procedure

Optimal positioning cannot be overemphasized; the lesion should be in the bottom half of the field; on occasion this entails repositioning the patient. Rigid proctoscopy in the operating room prior to positioning ensures correct patient position and minimizes the need for repositioning.

The Learning Curve

Much has been written recently about the leaning curve or the amount of time and/or number of procedures which need to be performed to achieve proficiency or expertise with a specified technique.

The learning curve has also been termed a "proficiency gain curve" [12] or the relationship between gaining experience with a technique and outcome variables such as operative time, complications, hospital stay, and mortality. In the case of TEM, the operative mortality should be almost nil and the hospital stay generally limited to an overnight stay, and thus outcome variables include technical ability to complete the excision with the TEM instruments and suture of the defect. The learning curve is steep in the beginning and should flatten with time and acquired expertise. Once expertise has been gained, the marginal improvement with each additional procedure is generally quite small.

Michel [12] has suggested that the learning cannot be confined simply to a learning curve and learning "is a process, not an event." He suggests that competence is not achieved once and for all, but involves a cyclical process evolving from incompetence to competence. With introduction of a new technology or technique, an individual passes from unconscious incompetence to awareness of his or her incompetence (conscious incompetence). Following a training period, the individual develops along the learning curve from conscious competence to unconscious competence where the steps of the procedure are ingrained or imprinted such that they are virtually automatic. At this point, however, the unconsciously competent individual needs to maintain his or her skill and be mindful of new techniques and procedures, lest he or she become unconsciously incompetent again.

Exactly how many procedures one needs to perform to have competence in the TEM procedure is not defined. In other procedures, such as laparoscopic colon resection for colon cancer, in a position statement the American Society of Colon and Rectal Surgeons and the Society of American Gastrointestinal Endoscopic Surgeons have suggested on the basis of the COST trial that an individual should have experience with at least 20 laparoscopic colorectal resections with anastomosis for benign disease or metastatic colon cancer before using the technique to treat curable cancer [13]. A surgeon should be proficient in techniques of transanal excision prior to embarking on the TEM procedure, but the number of procedures to gain competency is not known.

Conclusion

TEM is a safe, minimally invasive procedure for treatment of rectal polyps and selected rectal cancers. While the learning curve is steep, the superior optics and visualization and the ability to reach more proximal lesions have established TEM as an excellent option in selected patients. Proper training for both the surgeons and the operative team is essential to ensure successful development of a program in TEM. In addition, an adequate volume of appropriate cases is necessary to maintain a surgeon's skill and the proficiency of the operating room staff. Finally, wise "case selection" early on will ensure good outcomes, future referrals, and establishment of a successful TEM program.

References

1. Buess G, Gunther M. Endoscopic operative procedures for the removal of rectal polyps. *Coloproctology* 1984;6:254.
2. Saclarides TJ. Transanal endoscopic microsurgery. *Seminars in Laparoscopic Surgery* 2004;11:45–51.
3. Mellgren A, Sirivongs P, Rothenberger DA, Madoff RD, Garcia-Aquilar J. Is local excision adequate therapy for early rectal cancer? *Dis Colon Rectum* 2000;43(8):1064–71.
4. Sengupta S, Tjandra JJ. Local excision of rectal cancer: what is the evidence? *Dis Colon Rectum* 2001;44(9):1345–61.
5. Guillem JG, Chessin DB, Jeong SY, Kim W, Fogarty JM. Contemporary applications of transanal endoscopic microsurgery. *Clinical Colorectal Cancer* 2005;5(4):268–73.
6. Cataldo PA. Transanal endoscopic microsurgery. *Surg Clin N Am* 2006;86:915–925.
7. Casadesus D. Transanal endoscopic microsurgery: a review. *Endoscopy* 2006;38:418–423.
8. Saclarides TJ. Transanal endoscopic microsurgery:a single surgeon's experience. *Arch Surg* 1998;133:595–8.
9. Dafnis G, Pahlman L, Raa Y, Gustafsson UM, Graf W. Transanal endoscopic microsurgery:clinical and functional results. *Colorectal Disease* 2004:6:336–42.
10. Cataldo PA, O'Brien S, Osler T. Transanal endoscopic mircrosurgery: a prospective evaluation of functional results. *Dis Colon Rectum* 2005;48:1366–71.
11. Ganai S, Garb JL, Kanumuri P, Rao RS, Alexander AI, Wait RB. *J Gastrointest Surg* 2006;10:22–31.
12. Michel LA. The epistemology of evidence-based medicine. *Surg Endosc* 2007;21:145–51.
13. American Society of Colon and Rectal Surgeons. Position statement. Laparoscopic colectomy for curable cancer. Available at http://www.fascrs.org/displaycommon.cfm?an = 1&subarticlebr = 319: accessed March 3, 2007.

Chapter 6
Partial-Thickness Excision

Peter A. Cataldo and Neil J. Mortensen

Introduction

Transanal endoscopic microsurgery (TEM) facilitates excision of lesions throughout the entire rectum. Depending upon rectal location, full-thickness rectal wall excision can result in increased potential for complications. The proximal rectum, particularly anteriorly, is located within the peritoneal cavity, and wound dehiscence can lead to intraperitoneal sepsis. In women, the vagina is immediately anterior to the distal one third of the anterior rectum, putting patients at increased risk for anovaginal fistula following full-thickness resection. In the very distal rectum, just above the dentate line sphincter musculature is at risk, and full-thickness wounds heal poorly. In all these circumstances partial-thickness, or submucosal, excision is associated with lower morbidity. If the pathologic finding is appropriate (i.e., benign disease) partial-thickness rectal wall excision is an excellent alternative in these situations.

Indications

Partial-thickness excision is obviously not appropriate for malignant lesions, as by definition this will leave residual tumor within the rectal wall and lead to early local recurrence. Malignant rectal polyps should be included in the above category. Therefore, submucosal excision is limited to benign polypoid lesions confined to the rectal mucosa. Despite the limited list of indications, there are many large villous lesions amenable to partial-thickness TEM excision. Certain circumstances lend themselves particularly well to partial-thickness excision. Large carpeting villous adenomas frequently occupy significant portions of the rectal wall. Full-thickness excision and primary repair of the rectal defect will lead to closure under tension and/or luminal stenosis. In this situation, partial-thickness excision without closure eliminates these concerns. Very proximal benign lesions are often well above the peritoneal reflection particularly when located anteriorly in the rectum. Full-thickness excision is possible, but necessitates intraperitoneal entry. Closure of these defects can be difficult and intraperitoneal leakage can occur, leading to intra-abdominal sepsis. Partial-thickness excision eliminates these risks. Similarly, anterior rectal lesions in women abut the vaginal septum. Full-thickness excision can lead to inadvertent injury to the posterior

---

P.A. Cataldo
University of Vermont College of Medicine, Burlington, VT, USA

P.A. Cataldo, G.F. Buess (eds.), *Transanal Endoscopic Microsurgery*,
DOI 10.1007/978-0-387-76397-2_6, © Springer Science+Business Media, LLC 2009

vaginal wall, or wound closure can break down. Either circumstance can lead to rectovaginal fistula. These problems can be avoided with submucosal excision.

Finally, full-thickness excision wounds involving the proximal anal canal heal poorly, with higher rates of suture line dehiscence. This often leads to a prolonged, painful recovery, possibly with significant long-term functional consequences. Again, partial-thickness excision eliminates these risks.

Surgeons are correctly concerned about occult malignancy arising in large villous and tubular adenomas, making partial-thickness excision inadvisable. Reported rates vary from 2 to 40%. In many situations full-thickness excision is simple and safe and is clearly the procedure of choice. However, in the situations previously described, if the likelihood of malignancy is low, partialthickness excision may be the best option.

If prior biopsy reveals benign disease, intrarectal ultrasound reveals no submucosal invasion, and upon visual inspection (and palpation if possible) the lesion appears to be soft and nonulcerated, the likelihood of invasive carcinoma is very low. These masses can be excised in the submucosal plane. In the rare circumstance that occult malignancy is detected, either further TEM excision in the full-thickness plane, or radical resection can be performed as dictated by the final pathologic evaluation and anatomy. An additional benefit provided by this approach is that the extrarectal planes remain unviolated by the submucosal approach. Therefore, any difficulties in transabdominal, extrarectal dissection associated with prior full-thickness TEM are avoided.

Preoperative Preparation

Patients are prepared similarly to patients undergoing full-thickness TEM. The lesion must be visualized with flexible endoscopy and localized with rigid sigmoidoscopy to facilitate patient positioning in the operating room. Anorectal function should be evaluated. In most circumstances a careful history and detailed anal canal examination are all that is required. Comorbidities should be assessed and addressed as for any surgical procedure.

A complete mechanical and antibiotic bowel prep is performed the day prior to surgery. Intravenous antibiotics are given within 1 h of the operation and venous thromboembolism prophylaxis is instituted on the basis of perioperative risk assessment.

Operative Technique

The lesion location is confirmed prior to induction of anesthesia. Spinal or general anesthesia may be used. The patient is then positioned appropriately with the lesion oriented "toward the floor." For anterior lesions, patients are positioned prone with legs separated on "split-leg attachments," posterior lesions necessitate high lithotomy positioning, and lateral lesions either left or right lateral decubitus positioning with the hips flexed 90° and the knees fully extended to facilitate easy manipulation of the TEM instruments.

The anus is slowly dilated with three fingers and the operating proctoscope inserted. The lesion is localized to the lower half of the operative field and the scope fixed in place with the Martin arm. Appropriate connections are made and the rectum is insufflated.

When performing submucosal or partial-thickness TEM excision, infiltration with local anesthetic is often the key to success. Using a long needle (a gallbladder decompression needle from the laparoscopic cholecystectomy set works well), one very carefully injects

6 Partial-Thickness Excision

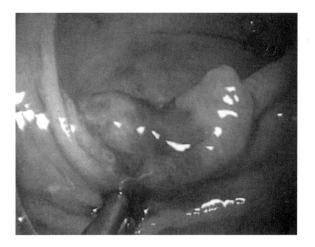

Fig. 6.1 Lidocaine with 1:100,000 epinephrine is injected in the submucosal plane, elevating the lesion off the underlying rectal musculature

1% lidocaine with 1:100,000 epinephrine just below the mucosa (Fig. 6.1). The entire lesion and 1-cm margins should be injected in this fashion. If the injection is in the correct plane, the lesion will clearly elevate off the underlying rectal wall. Proper injection will greatly facilitate excision in the correct plane. This point cannot be overemphasized.

Following injection, 1-cm margins are marked circumferentially around the mass to be excised with electrocautery using the fine needle tip (Fig. 6.2).

Dissection is begun distally and slowly in order to avoid entering the inner circular muscle layer of the rectal wall. Once the plane has been established, the distal margin (not the lesion) is grasped and elevated. This creates traction away from the underlying rectal wall and facilitates further dissection. If dissection is in the correct plane, the white, inner circular muscle fibers of the rectal wall will be clearly visible (Fig. 6.3).

Dissection continues circumferentially and deep to the lesion until the mass is entirely excised. Care should be taken to avoid dissection into the mucosa as this will "button-hole" the lesion and possibly result in incomplete excision. Occasionally, the dissection plane may penetrate the muscle or even the full-thickness rectal wall. If this occurs, the submucosal plane can be re-entered or the lesion excised in the full-thickness plane.

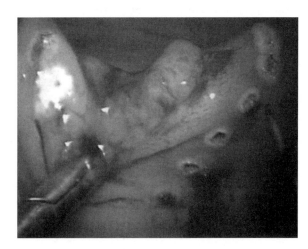

Fig. 6.2 One-centimeter margins are marked circumferentially around the polyp with electrocautery

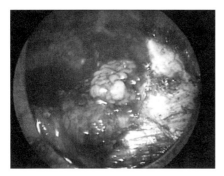 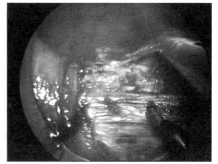

Fig. 6.3 The polyp has been partially dissected and is elevated off the rectal wall. The inner circular muscle fibers are visible deep to the plane of dissection

Fig. 6.4 Following submucosal excision, inner circular muscle fibers of the rectal wall are visible at the base of the resection defect

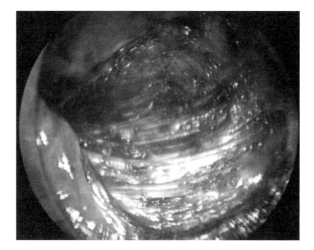

Once the mass has been excised, the site is inspected for bleeding and cauterized appropriately. A clear base of rectal muscle fibers will be visible (Fig. 6.4). The defect does not need to be sutured closed, but can be at the surgeon's discretion. Closure may slightly decrease postoperative bleeding risk. In addition, closing partial-thickness excision wounds increases a surgeon's experience, allowing him or her to become more facile with suturing techniques. This will lead to more secure defect closure in essential situations, such as intraperitoneal excisions.

Postoperative Care

The majority of patients undergoing partial-thickness TEM excision can be safely discharged directly from the postoperative care unit, or alternatively the day following surgery. With the exception of very distal lesions encroaching upon the dentate line, the procedure is often associated with remarkably little pain. Mild analgesics and a bowel regimen to prevent constipation are prescribed at the time of discharge.

The final pathologic evaluation is reviewed. If the lesion remains benign, no further treatment is necessary. Patients with positive resection margins and benign disease are carefully followed endoscopically for mucosal recurrence. If recurrence should develop, it is often small and can be resected colonoscopically. Repeat TEM excision is possible, but is rarely necessary. If the pathologic evaluation reveals malignancy, appropriate treatment is based once again on the pathologic findings in the patient's anatomy.

Complications

Complications following partial-thickness excision are rare. Bleeding is most common and often resolves with conservative treatment. Operative suture ligation with or without the aid of TEM instrumentation is rarely necessary, but can be performed for refractory hemorrhage. Sepsis, anovaginal fistula, and intraperitoneal infection are essentially unheard of following partial-thickness excision.

Conclusions

Partial-thickness or submucosal TEM resection is a useful tool for large benign rectal masses. Although occult malignancy must always be considered in large "benign" adenomatous lesions, visual inspection, ultrasound, and pathologic evaluation can minimize this risk in the majority of cases. Partial-thickness excision is particularly valuable for very proximal lesions, anterior masses adjacent to the anovaginal septum, and large lesions in the distal rectum.

References

1. Arebi N, Swain D, Suzuki N Fraser C, Price A, Saunders BP. Endoscopic mucosal resection of 161 cases of large sessile or flat colorectal polyps. Scand J Gastroenterol. 2007; 42(7):859–66.
2. Bach S, Lane L, Merrie A, Mortensen NJMcC. Stage 1 Rectal Cancer: transanal endoscopic microsurgery or radical resection. Colorectal Dis. 2006; 8:(Suppl 2) 19.
3. Bretagnol F, Merrie, A, George B, Warren BF, Mortensen NJ McC. Local excision of rectal tumours by transanal endoscopic microsurgery. Br J Surg. 2007; 94(5):627–33.
4. Hurlstone DP, Saunders DS, Cross SS, George R, Shorthouse AJ, Brown S. A prospective analysis of extended endoscopic mucosal resection for large rectal villous adenomas: an alternative technique to transanal endoscopic microsurgery. Colorectal Dis. 2005; 7(4):339–44.
5. McCloud JM, Waymont, N, Pahwa N, Vaarghese P, Richards C, Jameson JS, Scott AN. Factors predicting early recurrence after transanal endoscopic microsurgery excision for rectal adenoma. Colorectal Dis. 2006; 8(7):581–5.
6. Parks AG, Stuart AE. The management of villous tumours of the large bowel. Br J Surg. 1973 Sep; 60(9):688–95.
7. Steele RJ, Hershman, MJ, Mortensen NJMcC, Armitage NC, Scholefield JH. Transanal endoscopic microsurgery – initial experience from three centres in the United Kingdom. Br J Surg. 1996; 83(2):207–10.
8. Tamegai Y, Saito UY, Masaki N, Hinohara C, Oshima T, Kogure E, Liu Y, Uemura N, Saito K. Endoscopic submucosal dissection: a safe technique for colorectal tumours. Endoscopy. 2007; 39(5):418–22.
9. Whitehouse PA, Tilney HS, Armitage JN, Simson JN. Transanal endoscopic microsurgery: risk factors for local recurrence of benign rectal adenomas. Colorectal Dis. 2006; (9):795–9.

Chapter 7
Full-Thickness Excision

Emanuele Lezoche, Mario Guerrieri, Maddalena Baldarelli, and Giovanni Lezoche

Transanal endoscopic microsurgery (TEM) is a minimally invasive transanal surgical technique that uses a set of specialized endoscopic surgical instruments along with a form of enhanced or assisted vision (usually stereoscopic) to facilitate removal of tumors throughout the entire rectum.

The three-dimensional amplification, magnified stereoscopic view and lighting within the rectal lumen, with subsequent excellent vision of the operative field, allow the surgeon to perform extremely precise excision of rectal lesions, including full-thickness excision with perirectal fat and adjacent lymph nodes. This specific superiority also permits surgery for low rectal cancers with subsequent sphincter salvage.

The technique of TEM was first described and made available for clinical use in 1983 by Buess et al. in Germany. To our knowledge, this technique is currently the only one-port system which provides a completely endoluminal approach to the target organ using a natural opening of the body. TEM is primarily used for local excision of selected low, middle, and upper rectal tumors (both benign and selected malignant lesions). Consequently, patients may be able to avoid conventional surgery and to resume normal activities sooner. When used on appropriately selected early stage tumors, TEM can achieve oncologic results similar to those reported after radical resection, while limiting morbidity and mortality.

TEM may also be used for palliative purposes when patients have advanced disease and cure is unlikely, even with radical surgery.

Current Indications

1. Rectal adenomas (sessile polyps of the rectum)
2. Rectal carcinomas T1 well or moderately well differentiated (G1–G2)
3. Rectal carcinomas T1 poorly differentiated (G3) after neoadjuvant treatment
4. Rectal carcinomas T2–N0–M0 (smaller than 3 cm) after neoadjuvant treatment
5. Rectal carcinomas T3–N0–M0 (smaller than 3 cm) after significant response to neoadjuvant treatment
6. Rectal carcinomas independent of the stage as palliative treatment in high-risk patients for major surgery, or with a diffuse metastatic disease, or in patients who refused Miles operation

---

E. Lezoche
Dipartimento di Chirurgia Paride Stefanini, La Sapienza Universita' Di Roma, Policlinico Umberto I, Rome, Italy

P.A. Cataldo, G.F. Buess (eds.), *Transanal Endoscopic Microsurgery*,
DOI 10.1007/978-0-387-76397-2_7, © Springer Science+Business Media, LLC 2009

Preoperative Staging

Accuracy in the preoperative staging is mandatory to correctly select patients eligible for local excision. The routine use of the endorectal ultrasound combined with a computed tomography (CT) scan and magnetic resonance imaging (MRI) has revolutionized our ability to perform accurate preoperative staging with respect to rectal wall penetration (T stage), regional lymph nodes (N) and metastasis (M). Only patients who are lymph node negative, with tumor limited into the wall of the rectum, and with a diameter that does not exceed 3 cm should be considered eligible for local excision.

Techniques include:

1. Digital examination (to evaluate tumor fixation).
2. Total colonoscopy.
3. Rigid rectoscopy to

    – Perform macrobiopsies of the tumor area.
    – Measure the distance of the lesion from the anal verge.
    – Evaluate the circumferential position of the tumor.
    – Select appropriate patient surgical positioning.

4. Standard endoscopic biopsies of apparently normal mucosa are taken at a distance of 1 cm around the tumor, tattooed with India ink, and identified with a number (Fig. 7.1).
5. Transanal endosonography.
6. MRI or CT scan with 3-mm abdominal and pelvic sections (only for cancer).
7. Bone scintigraphy (only for cancer).
8. Chest X-ray (only for cancer).

Each macrobiopsy is examined by three different pathologists to assess the tumor grading. The parameters established for the grading are cellular differentiation (well, moderately well, or poor) and the lymphatic, blood vessel, and neural infiltration.

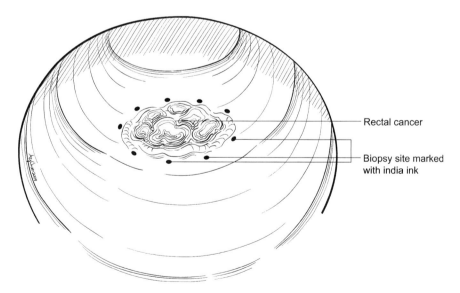

Fig. 7.1 Rectal cancer with circumferential biopsies 1 cm beyond visible tumor. Biopsy sites are marked with India ink

Neoadjuvant Therapy

Neoadjuvant therapy is indicated for T1 lesions with adverse histologic features, and for all T2 or T3 lesions. Two therapies are the radiotherapeutic options used before surgery. The first, called "short course," consists of the administration of a 15–25-Gy dose with single fractions of 5 Gy repeated for 3–5 days, followed 1 week later by surgical resection. The long course consists of 1.8–2.0-Gy fractions, five times a week for a total dose of 45 Gy; surgery is then performed 40 days following the completion of radiotherapy. The combination of radiotherapy with chemotherapy results in significant tumor mass reduction, which is particularly useful in association with local excision. The classic chemotherapy combination consists of mitomycin C in 1–29 days combined with 5-fluorouracil (5-FU) on days 1–4 and 29–32. The administration of cisplatin as a continuous infusion on days 1–29 combined with a continuous infusion of 5-FU on days 1–4 and 29–32 days is still under study. Randomized studies have demonstrated neoadjuvant therapy to be associated with a significant reduction in local recurrence and improved survival rates.

Neoadjuvant Therapy after Staging

For patients undergoing neoadjuvant therapy [T1 with cytologic and histologic high-risk features (G3) and for T2–T3 lesions], restaging is performed 40 days after completion of radiochemotherapy. Repeat staging of the rectal lesion consists of:

1. Digital examination
2. Endoscopy to evaluate the tumor diameter modification
3. Transanal ultrasound
4. MRI or CT scan with 3-mm abdominal and pelvic sections

Comparing the results of all these examinations with those performed preoperatively, we classify the effects of radiotherapy according to the T stage as follows. Cases are considered *downstaged* if all the imaging tests (ultrasound and CT scan or MRI) identify a lower T stage. When no downstaging is achieved we propose, according to our protocol, a classification of the tumor response (downsize) as follows: (1) *responders* if reduction of the tumor diameter is more than 50%; (2) *low responders* if diameter reduction is between 30 and 50%; (3) *non-responders* if diameter reduction is less than 30% or no reduction is observed.

Patient Preparation

The preoperative washout of the colon is performed the day before operation with 4 l of laxative with osmotic action (Selg-Esse 1000, Promefarm, Milan, Italy) and short-term antibiotic prophylaxis is applied.

Informed Consent

All patients have to be informed and have to sign a consent form concerning the oncologic risk of local excision, possible intraoperative and postoperative complications (bleeding, suture dehiscence, temporary gas or stool incontinence, conversion to laparotomy with colonic resection and colostomy, etc), and need for close postoperative follow-up when TEM is performed for malignant lesions.

Anesthesia

TEM is performed under general anesthesia in the majority of patients. In select high-risk patients (ASA 4) spinal anesthesia can be employed.

Instrumentation

The instrumentation described by Buess and produced by the Richard Wolf Company (Knittlingen, Germany) consists of a modified rectoscope 12 or 20 cm in length (external diameter of 4 cm) with three-dimensional vision and three operative channels. The lesion must be preoperatively localized by rigid rectoscopy and the patient consequently positioned in supine, lateral, or prone position in order to have the lesion placed in the inferior part of the operative field.

The rectoscope is fixed to the operative field by the Martin arm, a supporting instrument with two joints which maintain the optimal position of the rectoscope inside the rectum. The optical system consists of a three-dimensional 10-mm 50° stereoscope and a 5-mm 40° angled lens connected to a video system.

A multidimensional instrument (ICC 350, Erbe, Tuebingen, Germany) was developed in 1993 and consists of a device with four functions: bipolar high-frequency cutting, monopolar coagulation, suction, and irrigation. In the cutting mode, a pneumatically driven needle comes out from the lumen of the instrument; the current passes from the knife to the isolated metal ring at the distal end of the device, so that it functions as a bipolar high-frequency knife. In the coagulation mode, the knife is automatically withdrawn into the lumen and the metal ring can be used for monopolar coagulation. When bleeding is encountered in the operative field the knife of the combination device is retracted into a cannula and hemostasis is immediately performed using the monopolar coagulation ring.

In recent years two additional energy sources have become available:

1. Harmonic Scalpel (Ultracision, Johnson & Johnson Gateway), an ultrasonic cutting and coagulation surgical device
2. Electrothermal bipolar vessel sealing (EBVS; LigaSure, Atlas, Tyco Healthcare-USA)

A needle holder, forceps, and clip applicator are also utilized during the procedure. Water can be injected through the rectoscope to clean the lens and the operative field throughout the procedure. An endosurgically controlled CO_2-insufflation unit dilates the rectum with constant measurement of endoluminal pressure. The rectoscope is positioned so that the tumor is viewed "from above" at approximately 45°. After the operative rectoscope has been positioned, including the optics and surgical instruments, the resection begins by marking a 1–2-cm safety margin around the rectal tumor, using the coagulation mode of the multifunctional instrument (guided, in some cases, by Indian ink marks made previously). The three-dimensional view and use of the combination instrument allows for precise tumor excision at the previously demarcated safety margin.

Resection Options

- Mucosectomy involves removing the mucosa, including the polyp from the inner circular layer of the muscularis; a suitable technique for sessile adenomas located in the intraperitoneal portion of the rectum (Fig. 7.2a).
- Partial rectal wall excision consists of removal of a portion of the rectal wall separating the inner circular layer from the longitudinal muscle of the rectal wall (Fig. 7.2b).
- Full-thickness excision requires removal of all layers of the rectal wall in the plane just superficial to the perirectal fat. This is the excision performed for the majority of lesions localized in the extraperitoneal rectum. (Fig. 7.2c).
- Full-thickness excision with perirectal fat: a full-thickness excision including the adjacent perirectal fat containing lymph nodes is performed. This excision is indicated in cases of malignant lesions or very large polyps with suspected malignancy. For posterior lesions, the perirectal fat is removed, dissecting in the so-called holy plane outside the mesorectum. In the case of anterior tumors, the excision must reach the vaginal septum or the prostatic capsule. Once the excision is completed, the shape of the specimen is a "truncated pyramid" (Fig. 7.2d).

In cases of malignancy, the excision must always include a 1-cm margin of normal mucosa surrounding the lesion. It is of crucial importance to correctly orient the specimen on the cork board immediately after resection to evaluate the safety margins before fixation

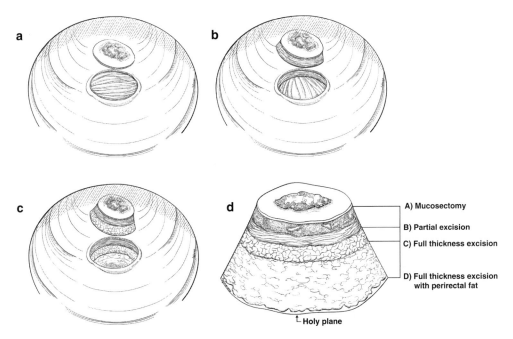

Fig. 7.2 a Mucosectomy. The benign tumor along with surrounding mucosa and submucosa are removed. The muscular rectal wall and perirectal fat are left in situ. **b** Partial rectal wall excision. The lesion and the mucosa, submucosa, and inner circular layer of the rectal wall are removed. **c** Full-thickness excision. The tumor and the entire thickness of the rectal wall are removed. **d** Segmental resection. When the lesion is circumferential, it is possible to perform a circumferential excision with subsequent complete end-to-end anastomosis

with formalin. The proximal and distal margins of resection have to be identified to ensure correct histologic examination.

The rectal defect is closed by running suture, transversely to prevent stenosis, with a polydioxanone (2/0) monofilament. The application of a silver clip at each end of the suture avoids the need for intraluminal suturing. Following excision of large masses, mobilization of the proximal and distal rectum well away from the rectal wall will minimize tension on the suture line. This maneuver, however, is rarely necessary. In addition, approximating large defects with a single suture at the midpoint places both the proximal and the distal margins adjacent to each other and facilitates closure. Following this, the defect is closed from the peripheral margins to the center in running fashion. For right-handed surgeons, it is easiest to close the right half of the excision with sutures placed from distal to proximal. Conversely, for the left side, sutures placed from proximal to distal facilitate closure. For defects occupying a significant percentage of the rectal circumference, it may be easier to use the straight (rather than angled) instruments when operating in the "upper-half" of the TEM visual field.

Perioperative Complications

Rare mortality is reported in the literature after TEM, whereas a morbidity about of 15% is common in most series.

Complications include:

1. *Bleeding*: The most frequent complication during operation is bleeding. In fact hemostasis is essential during dissection in endoscopic surgery. Without meticulous hemostasis, even minimal bleeding can obscure the view of the operative field. In this technique, in which the operator works in a very restricted space, quick and efficient hemostasis is vital for maintaining vision and avoiding unnecessary problems. The combination instrument for TEM allows the performance of hemostasis without changing instruments, as it can function both as a knife and as a suction and irrigation device. Additionally both the Harmonic Scalpel and EBVS (LigaSure) are beneficial in maintaining hemostasis.
2. *Intraperitoneal entry:* This in fact is not a complication of TEM, but a necessary occurrence when full-thickness excision of intraperitoneal rectal lesions is performed. When this occurs, pneumorectum is lost and exposure can be difficult. The patient should be placed in Trendelenburg position; this will prevent the small bowel from entering the rectal lumen. Careful exposure will often reveal the peritoneal edges. Reapproximation of the peritoneum will re-establish rectal distention and allow for safe closure of the rectal wall in a separate layer. Occasionally, it will not be possible to close the peritoneum separately. In this circumstance, a careful, single, full-thickness closure of the rectal defect is appropriate. Following closure of the intraperitoneal rectum, some surgeons will perform a water-soluble contrast enema on postoperative day 1 prior to beginning oral intake.
3. *Fistula*: In women, if the lesion is located in the anterior wall of the rectum, the possibility of rectovaginal fistula exists. Careful gentle, blunt dissection of the rectovaginal septum must be performed, avoiding eletrocoagulation. It may be beneficial for the surgeon to place a finger in the vagina to confirm normal anatomy. If the injury is recognized during TEM it can easily be repaired. The vagina and the rectum should be closed in separate layers. If possible, the two suture lines should not be directly on top of

one another. If the fistula resides in the very distal rectum, then removal of the TEM equipment and closure with standard transanal techniques is also an option.

If the fistula is unrecognized, or develops postoperatively (often owing to excessive use of electrocautery), it should be repaired at a later date when all inflammation has resolved. In men during the dissection of the prostatic capsule, electrocoagulation must be employed to avoid of bleeding from the prostatic vessels. During wide dissection a small urethral lesion may rarely occur but can be easily sutured. In this circumstance, a urethral catheter should be left in place for 2 weeks postoperatively. A urethrogram documenting successful healing is obtained at the time of catheter removal.

4. *Suture line disruption:* Intraperitoneal suture line disruption results in pelvic peritonitis. This complication often requires transabdominal drainage with or without proximal diversion, depending upon the size of the leak, the degree of contamination, and the clinical status of the patient. Primary closure of the defect is rarely successful owing to local inflammation. In a delayed leak with localized abscess formation, CT-guided percutaneous drainage may be indicated.

Extraperitoneal leaks present with rectal pain, drainage, and fever. In many cases these respond to antibiotics combined with local analgesic enemas. Occasionally examination under anesthesia and drainage (often opening the remaining suture line) may be necessary.

5. *Incontinence:* The considerable diameter of the rectoscope can cause temporary stool incontinence; generally symptoms resolve within 2 months following surgery. Despite the considerable anal stretch by the rectoscope, anorectal function does not seem to be significantly impaired by the TEM procedure and generally returns to normal within a few months.

In order to limit the sphincter damage we recommend the following:

- Before introducing the rectoscope a smooth dilatation of the sphincter must be performed slowly (at least in 5 min) and tearing must be avoided.
- Operative time should be less than 90 min, if possible, as the rectoscope inside the anal canal may induce a reduction of the blood supply to the muscular fibers. Longer operations have been associated with higher rates of incontinence.
- During the operation the main axis of the rectoscope should remain as parallel as possible to the anal canal axis. Increases in this angle result in further dilatation of the anal sphincter and subsequent possible sphincter injury.
- Avoid posterior compression of the sphincter fibers between the rectoscope and the coccyx.

Resection Margins

In patients undergoing preoperative chemoradiotherapy, to ensure correct rectal tumor margins, we suggest the strategy of tattooing biopsy sites 1 cm around the tumor in order to identify the exact limits of the neoplasia (see point 4 in "Preoperative Staging", Fig. 7.1). This approach is important when lesions dramatically decrease in size or disappear after chemoradiotherapy. Once the specimen has been removed, we suggest further removal of a second full-thickness semicircular margin of 0.5 cm in length both in the oral and the aboral margin of the incision (Fig. 7.3). In addition, According to our experience we strongly recommend routine application of "a vital dye" for benign and malignant lesions. This may reveal subtle areas of residual adenoma that may be responsible for local recurrence or become malignant with time.

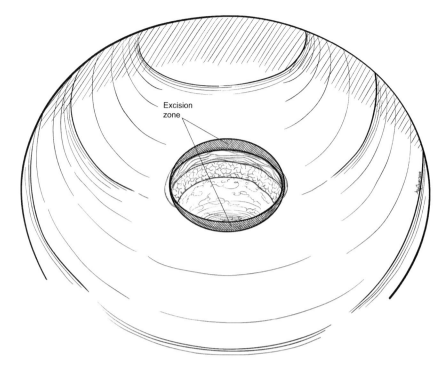

Fig. 7.3 Additional 1-cm proximal and distal resection margins are excised following section of malignant lesion to ensure tumor-free margins

TEM for Rectal Cancer

Twenty five years after the introduction of the total mesorectal excision by Heald, many surgeons perform this operation in all stages of rectal cancer despite the fact there is no scientific evidence that proves the value of total mesorectal excision in nonadvanced rectal cancer (T2N0Mx). Low anterior resection has significant postoperative morbidity, and in high-risk patients perioperative mortality ranges between 1 and 5%. Urinary and sexual sequelae and permanent stomas are other factors that significantly impair quality of life after surgery for low rectal cancer. In 1992, we originated a clinical protocol for selected T2 and T3 N0 rectal cancer with the aim of developing a diagnostic and therapeutic algorithm to select patients with nonadvanced rectal cancer eligible for local excision by TEM. The goal was to obtain oncologic results equal to those of radical surgery while avoiding the high rate of postoperative complications, mortality, and functional sequelae.

Timing of Neoadjuvant Therapy

Neoadjuvant treatment is universally accepted for advanced rectal cancer. Since 1992 we have employed radiotherapy in T2 and T3 lesions to obtain better local control of the disease. In our experience all patients (including high-risk ones) were able to complete a full course of high-dose radiotherapy. Since 1997, patients have followed a protocol that includes continuous infusion of 200 mg/m^2/day 5-FU administered throughout radiotherapy.

For T1 rectal cancer, the percentage of nodal involvement ranges from 0 to 12% (about 3% in T1 lesions with a favorable histologic grade and 12% in T1 lesions with a poor prognostic grade). On the basis of these data, in recent years, we have routinely employed neoadjuvant treatment for patients staged preoperatively as T1 with cytologic and histologic and high-risk features (G3).

The Stockholm I and II randomized trials have definitively established the advantage of preoperative radiotherapy in preventing local failure and today there is general agreement in the literature that preoperative radiochemotherapy results in significant tumor downstaging, better local control of the disease, and may improve also the overall survival, particularly in advanced rectal cancer. Neoadjuvant therapy may result in tumor mass reduction, resulting in a less destructive surgery with decreased postoperative complications rates and with sphincter preservation. Other potential advantages are radiation is delivered to well-oxygenated tissue, eradication of the local regional micrometastatic disease, and reduction of intraoperative local or distant dissemination of neoplastic cells.

There are two radiotherapeutic options available before surgery: the first, called "short course", consists of the administration of a 15–25-Gy dose with single fractions of 5 Gy repeated for 3–5 days, followed by surgery; the second consists of 1.8–2.0-Gy sessions, five times a week for a total dose that varies from 35 to 45 Gy; surgery is done 40 days after the completion of radiotherapy. With both techniques, randomized studies have demonstrated a significant reduction of local recurrence.

The 40-day course, since it provides more time for downstaging, can expand the indications for local excision. For these reasons we prefer to utilize the standard course of radiotherapy (4,500 cGy) combined with chemotherapy and surgery 40 days after the end of the neoadjuvant treatment, in order to avoid tissue edema and to obtain the most significant tumor mass reduction. Furthermore, the fibrosis induced by long-term radiotherapy seems to be more effective in destroying lymphatic and venous vessels, reducing the risk of lymphovascular spread of neoplastic cells during surgical manipulations. In addition, in cases of advanced incurable rectal cancer neoadjuvant therapy can be combined with palliative TEM.

Lymph Node Sampling

Recently we have employed in vivo lymphoscintigraphy to ensure removal of all the lymphatic tissue draining the tumor. We have used a modified sentinel lymph node technique in all patients undergoing preoperative radiotherapy. Forty minutes before the operation, we inject the submucosa under the tumor and 1 cm peripheral margins with ^{99m}Tc-labeled particles of nanocolloid (10 MBq) in 0.2 ml. The radiotracer diffuses though the lymphatic tissues, reaching the lymph nodes in the lymphatic drainage basin. TEM procedure is then carried out and once the lesion has been removed it is evaluated with the aid of a gamma probe (Scinti probe MR 100 Pol. Hi. Tec.) to identify any areas of high activity. In these cases the radioactive source is sent to the pathologist for intraoperative examination. Then the probe is reintroduced into the rectum through the rectoscope and all margins of the excision are carefully checked to identify any areas of residual activity. These sites are marked with metallic clips; then the TEM optic is reinserted into the rectoscope and resection of all the areas identified is performed. At the end of the procedure, the probe is reinserted to verify all the radioactive areas have been completely removed.

TEM in Rectal Cancer: State of the Art

The recent literature reports that local excision is curative in patients with a primary tumor which is limited to the mucosa and the submucosa without high-risk features (poor differentiation, vascular and neural invasion, presence of mucinous structures, and tumor ulceration) as clearly stated in guidelines for treatment of colon and rectal cancer (National Comprehensive Cancer Network, version IV, February 2005).

In 1996, Winde et al. reported the results of a prospective randomized trial that compared T1N0 rectal cancer treated by TEM versus anterior resection. That study clearly showed no statistically significant difference in local recurrence (4.2%) and 5-year survival rates (96%). In contrast, significant differences were found in the group of patients undergoing local excision by TEM in terms of length of hospitalization, loss of blood, analgesic use, and early and late morbidity. Winde et al. concluded that for early rectal cancer (T1N0), TEM was preferred because of lower morbidity with a similar percentage of local recurrence and survival rates.

Recently we have reported the results of TEM in 100 patients with small s T2–T3–N0–M0 distal rectal cancer after preoperative high-dose radiotherapy. The probability of local failure at the end of follow-up (10 years) was 5% and the probability of metastasis was 2%. The rectal cancer specific survival rate at the end of follow-up (10 years) was 89% and the overall survival was 72%. These results are not significantly different from those obtained in our experience after radical or laparoscopic surgery.

Many criticisms of this study are related to the fact that it was not a randomized trial and that these were selected patients. Therefore, we decided to perform a prospective randomized trial, which is still ongoing. Inclusion criteria are: patients staged at admission as T2N0, tumor located within 6 cm from the anal verge, tumor diameter less than 3 cm, lymph node negative (N0), and no signs of systemic or metastatic disease.

Following chemoradiotherapy, patients are randomized for laparoscopic radical resection or TEM. Preliminary results have identified similar local recurrence rates and overall survival for both groups. At present, despite the favorable long-term results, we still limit local excision to a select group of patients with T2 and T3 rectal cancer, and before drawing any further conclusions we will wait for the results of other randomized trials.

Conclusions

In conclusion, we can affirm that TEM is a minimally invasive technique which allows precise excision of tumors throughout the entire rectum via a transanal approach. Compared with the traditional transanal approach using Park's retractor, TEM achieves better exposure of the operative field with rectal distention and stereoscopic magnified endoscopic vision. The precise excision of the tumor obtained by TEM facilitates a more accurate and oncologically sound operation. Literature reports have proven the benefits of local excision, including decreased surgical trauma, sphincter preservation, reduction in perioperative complications, and faster postoperative recovery. Oncologic results are promising for select rectal cancers, but definitive recommendations await the results of further prospective, randomized trials.

Selected References

Balch GC, De Meo A, Guillem JG. Modern management of rectal cancer. A 2006 update. *World J Gastroenterol* 2006,12:3186–3195.

Blair S, Ellenhorn JD. Transanal excision for low rectal cancers is curative in early-stage disease with favorable histology. *Am Surg* 2000 Sept.;66 (9):817–20.

Bosset JF, Magnin V, Maigon P, et al. Preoperative radiochemotherapy in rectal cancer: Long-term results of a phase in trial. *Int J Rad Onc Biol Phys* 2000;46:323–327.

Bozzetto F, Baratti D, Andreola S, Zucali R, Schiavo M, Spinelli P, Gronchi A, Bertario L, Mariani L, Gennari L. Preoperative radiation therapy for patients with T2-T3 carcinoma of the middle-to-lower rectum. *Cancer* 1999;86:398–404.

Buess GF, Raestrup H. Transanal endoscopic microsurgery. *Surg Oncol Clin N Am.* 2001 July;10 (3):709–731.

Buess G, Mentges B. Transanal Endoscopic Microsurgery (T.E.M.). *Minimally Invasive Therapy* 1992;1:101–9.

Cedemark B, Johansson H, Rutqvist L.E, Wilking N, et al. The Stockholm I trial of preoperative short term radiotherapy in operable rectal carcinoma. *Cancer* 1995;75:2269–2275.

Chakravarti A, Compton CC, Shellito PC, Wood WC, Landry J, Machuta SR, Kaufman D, Ancukiewicz M, Willett CG. Long-term follow-up of patients with rectal cancer managed by local excision with and without adjuvant irradiation. *Ann Surg* 1999 July;230 (1):49–54.

Dahl O, Horn A, Morild I, et al. Low dose preoperative radiation postpones recurrences in operable rectal cancer. Results of a randomized multicenter trial in western Norway. *Cancer* 1990;66:2286–94.

Graham RA, Hackford AW, Wazer DE. Local excision of rectal carcinoma: a safe alternative for more advanced tumors? *J Surg Oncol* 1999 Apr;70 (4):235–38.

Grann A, Minsky BD, Cohen AM, et al. Preliminary results of preoperative 5-fluorouracil, low dose leucovorin and concurrent radiation therapy for resectable T3 rectal cancer. *Dis Colon Rectum* 1997;40:515–522.

Gerard A, Buyse M, Nordlinger B, et al. Preoperative radiotherapy as adjuvant treatment in rectal cancer. Final results of a randomized study of the European Organization for Research and Treatment cancer (EORTC). *Ann Surg* 1988;208:606–614.

Goldberg PA, Nicholls RJ, Porter NH, et al. Long-term results of a randomized trial of short-course low-dose adjuvant preoperative radiotherapy for rectal cancer. Reduction in local treatment failure. *Eur J Cancer* 1994;30A:1602–1606.

Habr-Gama A, Perez RO, Kiss DR, Rawet V, Scanavini A, Santinho PM, Nadalin W. Preoperative chemoradiation therapy for low rectal cancer. Impact on downstaging and sphincter-saving operations. *Hepatogastroenterology* 51:1703–1707.

Heintz A, Morschel M, Junginger T. (1998) Comparison of results after transanal endoscopic microsurgery and radical resection for T1 carcinoma of the rectum. *Surg Endosc* 12:1145–1148.

Heald RJ (1995) Total mesorectal excision is optimal surgery for rectal cancer: a Scandinavian consensus. *Br J Surg* 82;10:1297–1299.

Kapiteijn E, Marijnen CA, Nagtegaal ID, Putter H, Steup WH, Wiggers T, Rutten HJ, Pahlman L, Glimelius B, van Krieken JH, Leer JW, van de Velde CJ. Dutch Colorectal Cancer Group. Preoperative radiotherapy combined with total mesorectal excision for respectable rectal cancer. *N Engl J Med* 2001;345 (9):638–46.

Kim CJ, Yeatman TJ, Coppola D, Trotti A, Williams B, Barthel JS, Dinwoodie W, Karl RC, Marcet J. Local excision of T2 and T3 rectal cancers after downstaging chemoradiation. *Ann Surg* 2001;234 (3):352–58. Discussion 358–59.

Lee W, Lee D, Choi S, Chun H. Transanal endoscopic microsurgery and radical surgery for T1 and T2 rectal cancer. *Surg Endosc* 2003;17;1283–87.

Lezoche E, Guerrieri M, Paganini AM, Feliciotti F, Di Pietrantonj F. Is transanal endoscopic microsurgery (TEM) a valid treatment for rectal tumors? *Surg Endosc* 1996;10:736–41.

Lezoche E., Guerrieri M, Paganini AM, Baldarelli M, De Sanctis A, Lezoche G. Long-Term Results in Patients with T2-T3-N0 Distal Rectal Cancer Submitted to Radiotherapy Prior to Transanal Endoscopic Microsurgery. *Br J Surg* 2005, Dec.;92 (12):1546–52.

Lezoche E, Guerrieri M, Paganini AM, D'Ambrosio G, Baldarelli M, Lezoche G, Feliciotti F, De Sanctis A. Transanal endoscopic microsurgery versus total mesorectal laparoscopic resections of T2-N0 low rectal cancer after neoadjuvant treatment: a prospective randomized trial with a 3 years minimum follow-up period. *Surg Endosc* 2005;19:751–756.

Martling AL, Holm T, Rutqvist LE, Moran BJ, Heald RJ, Cedemark B. (2000) Effect of surgical training programme on outcome of rectal cancer in the County of Stockholm. Stockholm Colorectal Cancer Study Group, Basingstoke Bowel Cancer Research Project. *Lancet* 356:93–6.

Marijnem CA, Glimelius B. (2002) The role of radiotherapy in rectal cancer. *Eur J Cancer* 38:943–952.

Marks G, Mohiuddin M, Masoni L. The reality of radical sphincter preservation surgery for rectal of the distal 3 cm of rectum following high-dose radiation. *Int J Radiat Oncol Biol Phys* 1993;27:779–83.

Marks G, Mohiuddin M, Rakinic J. New hope and promise for sphincter preservation in the management of cancer of the rectum. *Semin Oncol* 1991;18:88–98.

Marks G, Mohuiddin M, Masoni L, Pecchioli L. High-dose preoperative radiation and full-thickness local excision. A new option for patients with select cancers of the rectum. *Dis Colon Rectum* 1990;33:735–39.

Marsh PJ, James RD, Schofield PF, et al. Adjuvant preoperative radiotherapy for locally advanced rectal carcinoma. Results of a prospective randomized trial. *Dis Colon Rectum* 1994;37:1205–1214.

Mentges B, Buess G, Effinger G, Manncke K, Becker HD. Indications and results of local treatment of rectal cancer. *Br J Surg* 1997;84:348–351.

Navarro M, Perez F, Cotor EM, et al. Preoperative chemoradiotherapy in locally advanced rectal cancer. Preliminary results (Abst). Proc Ann Meet ASCO, 2000;19:A313.

Rodel C, Martus P, Papadoupolos T, Fuzesi L, Klimpfinger M, Fietkau R, Hohenberger W, Raab R, Sauer R, Wittekind C. (2005) Prognostic Significance of tumor regression after chemoradiotherapy for rectal cancer. *J Clin Oncol* 23;8688–896.

Rouanet P, Fabre JM, Dubois JB, et al. Conservative surgery for low rectal carcinoma after high-dose radiation. *Ann Surg* 1995;221:67–73.

Ruo L, Guillem JG, Minsky BD, Quan SH, Paty PB, Cohen AM. (2002) Preoperative radiation with or without chemotherapy and full-thickness transanal excision for selected T2 and T3 distal rectal cancers. *Int J Colorectal Dis* 17:54–58.

Sengupta S, Tjandra JJ. Local excision of rectal cancer: what is the evidence? *Dis Colon Rectum* 2001 Sept.; 44 (9):1345–61.

Shirouzu K, Isomoto H, Kakegawa T. Distal spread of rectal cancer and optimal distal margin of resection for sphincter-preserving surgery. *Cancer* 1995 Aug 1; 76 (3):388–92.

Tanaka S, Kaltenbach T, Chayama K, Soetikno R. High-magnification colonoscopy (with videos). *Gastrointestinal Endoscopy* 2006;64:604–613.

Vecchio FM, Valentini V, Minsky BD, Padula GD, Venkatraman ES, Balducci M, Micciche F, Ricci R, Morgani AG, Gambacorta MA, Maurizi F. Coco C. The relationship of pathologic tumor regression grade (TRG) and outcomes after preoperative therapy in rectal cancer. *Int J Radiat Oncl Biol Phys* 2005;62:752–760.

Winde G, Nottberg H. Keller R, Schmid KW, Bunte H. Surgical cure for early rectal carcinomas (T1). Transanal Endoscopic microsurgery vs. anterior resection. *Dis Colon Rectum* 1996;39:969–976.

Chapter 8
Advanced Surgical Techniques

Prakash Gatta and Lee L. Swanstrom

Introduction

Transanal endoscopic microsurgery (TEM) has been utilized as a minimally invasive approach for low rectal lesions for over two decades. The primary indications are resection of suspicious or nonendoscopically resectable rectal polyps, early cancers or rectal ulcers. Surgeons who include TEM as a part of their practice can relate to the rather steep learning curve associated with performing this surgery for even basic resections. However, once over the learning curve, the surgeon can use TEM for a variety of more complex transanal procedures. Such advanced procedures include extended full-thickness excision, rectal sleeve resection, transanal fistula closure and, finally, TEM as a portal for natural orifice transluminal endoscopic surgery (NOTES). With the limitation of workspace within the rectum, performing more advanced procedures by TEM presents a formidable challenge to the surgeon. The surgeon should be very facile with basic TEM skills, particularly suturing. All advanced cases have the possibility of requiring either conversion to open, or laparoscopic procedures, or the need for flexible endoscopy. It is necessary to have available equipment and the skills to use when undertaking advanced TEM operations. With this, TEM can be a safe alternative to a wide variety of open and laparoscopic rectal procedures.

Indications and Patient Selection

Extended Full-Thickness Resection

There is particular concern about the appropriate treatment of rectal cancers; particularly the adequacy of resection margins and accurate staging when performing local resection. The magnification and exposure offered by TEM has been demonstrated to be an excellent property to achieve clear lateral margins, but concern remains regarding the deep margins and the status of local lymph nodes. Elective transanal resections for patients who are otherwise good candidates for a curative laparoscopic or open rectal resection therefore remain controversial. Lezoche et al. [1] recently reported 3-year outcomes of a prospective randomized trial comparing TEM with laparoscopic resection of T2 N0 rectal cancers following neoadjuvant chemotherapy. Their findings demonstrated comparable results between the two arms and less operative morbidity for the TEM

L.L. Swanstrom (✉)
Minimally Invasive Surgery, Legacy Health System and Oregon Clinic, Portland, OR, USA

P.A. Cataldo, G.F. Buess (eds.), *Transanal Endoscopic Microsurgery*,
DOI 10.1007/978-0-387-76397-2_8, © Springer Science+Business Media, LLC 2009

patients. The study concluded that TEM full-thickness excision of rectal cancer may be considered safe in patients having T2 N0 tumors, treated in conjunction with neoadjuvant chemoradiotherapy. They stressed the need for an extended full-thickness resection when performing TEM in order to achieve clear deep margins and for accurate cancer staging. We also feel that if TEM is offered as an alternative to formal rectal resection for known or suspected cancers, it is advisable to perform an extended deep resection. In most circumstances, patients with lesions greater than uT2 depth of invasion or having suspicious lymphadenopathy are not considered candidates for curative transanal resection. We describe below an extensive deep resection to remove the perirectal fat and lymph nodes in continuity with the specimen for early cancers.

In the past, surgeons have been cautious about performing aggressive full-thickness resections above the peritoneal reflection, often describing lesions above 15 cm as a contraindication to TEM in spite of the fact that the TEM instrumentation allows resection and closure up to 24 cm from the anus. It is our experience, however, that aggressive full-thickness resection can be safely performed even when it involves entrance into the peritoneal cavity [2]. Such resections require meticulous technique particularly with respect to closure of the rectotomy.

Sleeve Resection

Rectal sleeve resection has been advocated for procedures including rectovaginal fistulae, large circumferential polyps and rectal prolapse [3, 4]. Despite being technically difficult, sleeve resection can be performed using the improved visualization and precision of TEM. Although proof of reduced postoperative complications remains to be determined, TEM offers the theoretical advantage of more accurate suturing and therefore a reduced leak rate.

Rectal Fistulae

In the setting of rectal fistulae, the role of TEM can be considered less ambiguous. In addition to the clear superiority of identification and repair of fistulae, TEM may have the added benefit of better preservation of sphincter function. Ideal indications are mature rectovaginal, rectourethral, colovesicular and enterocolic fistulae below 22 cm. Contraindications include complex fistula disease such as Crohn's rectal disease, acute infections and fistula associated with rectal stricturing.

Transanal Intraabdominal Endoscopic Surgery

NOTES has generated interest for potential transgastric approaches to the peritoneum, sparing patients the morbidity of any abdominal wall incisions. Franklin et al. [11] has described the use of the rectal stump for removal of resected colon specimens during laparoscopic colon surgery—thereby avoiding creation of a large specimen removal site. This experience has given rise to the concept of using a rectotomy as an access point to intraperitoneal organs; essentially performing incisionless abdominal surgery. We propose that TEM technology may be an ideal platform for transrectal NOTES. TEM can be used

8 Advanced Surgical Techniques

to provide a secure "gateway" for such surgery, permitting easy access to the rectotomy for a variety of scopes and instruments, utilizing the proven ability of TEM to safely close the rectotomy

Surgeon Selection

Performing advanced procedures is recommended only for surgeons facile with routine TEM resections. Advanced laparoscopy skills (and availability of laparoscopic instrumentation) as well as flexible endoscopic skills are important. Although there have been no randomized controlled studies on outcomes, we have postulated 20 polypectomies to be an adequate number before progressing to more advanced procedures. Needless to say, only surgeons experienced enough to manage possible postoperative complications such as leaks and fistulae should incorporate this as part of their practice and surgeons should always be prepared to convert these advanced cases to a laparoscopic, or even an open, procedure.

Instrumentation

The most common TEM equipment is manufactured by Richard Wolf of Germany. Equipment employed includes a 12- or 20-cm beveled operating proctoscope. The proctoscope comes equipped with a glass faceplate for initial localization of the lesion and positioning of the proctoscope. After appropriate positioning of the device, the faceplate is removed and replaced with a sealed silicone faceplate which has four ports. The proctoscope is fixed to the operating table using the U-shaped arm provided. This arm can be loosened by the surgeon to adjust positioning of the scope during the operation if necessary. Surgeons may use either a direct viewing stereoscopic setup or an adapter which allows a standard laparoscope to be used. We prefer to use the 10-mm, 30° laparoscope for its easily availability and familiarity to operating room staff. It also allows the entire operating staff to see the procedure in real time on additional video monitors. Surgeons unfamiliar with laparoscopic setup and visualization may find the stereoscopic setup more helpful although it is less ergonomic [5]. The operation may be performed with special angled TEM instruments, although standard laparoscopic instruments are often used as well. Insufflation is maintained by Wolf's Laparo-CO2-Pneumo and TEM pump combination unit, which maintains pneumorectum while applying continual suction to prevent overdistention and to evacuate smoke.

Preoperative Workup

Every patient should have a complete screening colonoscopy and patients with a suspected rectal lesion require a preoperative rectal ultrasound examination. The location and proximity to the anus are determined in the preoperative workup to help determine patient positioning during the case. In patients with rectal cancer, a CT scan of the abdomen and pelvis is obtained to rule out advanced local or metastatic disease. Most patients with uT2 cancers are sent for evaluation for neoadjuvant chemotherapy prior to the operation. A standard cardiopulmonary assessment should be made to ensure that the patient is an acceptable candidate for general or regional anesthesia.

Patient Preparation

Potential TEM patients need to be extensively counseled before surgery as they may have unrealistic expectations regarding TEM. They should particularly be told about complication rates, including infections, abscesses, strictures, fistulae and leak risk (1%). Other complications include transient and rarely permanent fecal incontinence, postoperative bleeding and diarrhea. All patients are instructed to report any postoperative fevers or persistent bleeding or diarrhea. They should also be made aware of the possibility of abandoning the procedure or converting to a laparoscopic approach.

Patients undergoing TEM for rectal cancer should be aware that multiple treatment options exist, and that recurrence rates vary. Some surgeons believe radical, transabdominal resection should be performed for all rectal cancers regardless of the stage. Others believe local excision is appropriate for select, early cancers. The exact role of adjuvant (preoperative or postoperative) chemoradiotherapy remains unknown. Patients may require a second, radical resection following TEM if more advanced disease is identified on pathologic evaluation (i.e., T3 or N1) or if resection margins are involved with tumor.

All patients are placed on a clear liquid diet prior to surgery and given a standard oral phospha-soda prep the night before. A second-generation cephalosporin antibiotic is administered intravenously 30 min before the start of the surgery. Prophylaxis against deep venous thrombosis is critical as advanced TEM procedures can be lengthy and the patient's position often is not conducive to venous return. Pneumatic compression devices are applied to the legs and prophylaxis with low molecular weight heparin should be considered, particularly in patients with malignancy.

Technique

Extended Full-Thickness Resection

Specific Indications

Current indications include uT1 or uT2 rectal cancers or large tubulovillous adenomas involving less than one third of the circumference of the rectum. Ideal locations are in the middle or upper third of the rectum, although lower-third lesions are not a contraindication. All patients with suspected pT2 lesions are sent first for neoadjuvant therapy. Local resection is for cure contraindicated in pT3 lesions, unless comorbidities prohibit radical resection or the patient refuses an operation resulting in a permanent colostomy.

Room Preparation

All surgeries are performed under general anesthesia. Patient positioning depends on the location of the lesion as determined by initial workup. Rigid sigmoidoscopy is done prior to initiating TEM to confirm the location of the lesion. A Foley catheter is placed for all patients having an extended resection. A fully trained operating room staff familiar with the complex TEM equipment is critical to the efficient undertaking of each case. The TEM insufflator is placed either on designated laparoscopic towers or on a cart of its own to allow for easy movement of equipment in and out of a room. The insufflator is placed in clear view of the surgeon to help in effective troubleshooting if necessary. The operation is best performed in designated minimally invasive surgery (MIS) suites equipped with movable flat screen monitors and recording facilities. This allows the circulating nurse to have a monitor of his or her own to efficiently follow progress of the operation. The surgeon typically operates seated with the assistant at the left to wash the laparoscope lens as needed, alter the degree of the angled laparoscope and provide suction. The primary monitor is placed over the patient's torso directly in front of the surgeon.

Procedure

The patient is placed on a beanbag and positioned according to the location of the lesion to be resected. Whenever possible the patient is positioned in high lithotomy position, which is the easiest and most ergonomic (Fig. 8.1). Lithotomy position provides excellent exposure to posterior lesions and, because of its convenience, is often used for smaller lateral or even anterior lesions. However with the most commonly used beveled operating proctoscope, access to more anterior lesions is difficult in the lithotomy position. Therefore, anterior lesions are resected with the patient in the prone position (Fig. 8.2), and complex lateral lesions are resected with the patient in the lateral or "fetal" position (Fig. 8.3).

The patient is therefore positioned accordingly on a beanbag with lower extremities well padded. The proctoscope is inserted and advanced with the clear faceplate attached to allow for quick localization and centralization of the target. The most commonly used proctoscope is of 12-cm length (for lesions less than 15 cm from the anal verge) and the 20-cm-long proctoscope is reserved for higher rectal lesions as it is more difficult to suture through. Once positioning is satisfactory, the proctoscope is fixed to the operating table using the U-shaped arm. This arm can be manipulated easily during the operation if the operating field needs to be modified.

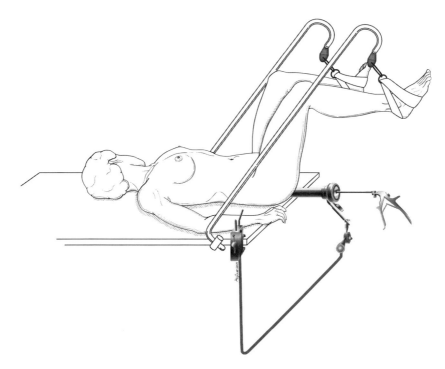

Fig. 8.1 Patient positioned supine in high lithotomy position for posterior lesions

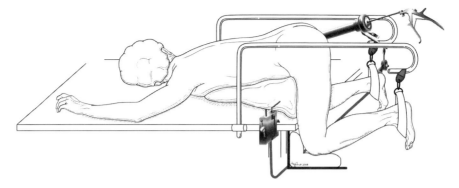

Fig. 8.2 Patient positioned prone for anterior lesions

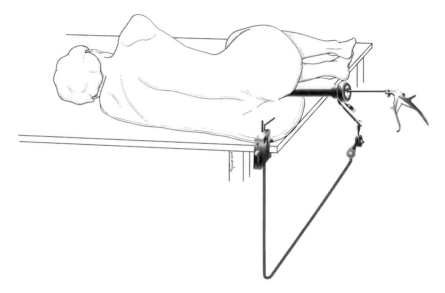

Fig. 8.3 "Fetal" position for lateral lesions

Wide margins of resection (at least 1 cm) are carefully marked circumferentially, using an angled needle cautery. Wider margins are used for known cancers. The marks are approximately 1 cm apart. The submucosal and perirectal planes are injected using diluted epinephrine solution to aid in hemostasis. A monopolar needle cautery at a standard electrocautery setting is used for the resection. The marks are used to outline the lesion and then are connected, dividing the rectal wall perpendicular to the mucosa. The mucosa is divided using the cutting function of the cautery and coagulation or "blend" setting is used for deeper tissues. The submucosal plane is the most vascular plane and the continuous suction probe is used to maintain adequate visualization. The layers of the rectal wall are divided perpendicular to the mucosa to maintain full-thickness margins, making the incision deep into the perirectal fat. When possible one should create the proximal incision early to prevent undermining during the deep dissection. As opposed to a known benign lesion, where a simple flap is elevated, the dissection is continued perpendicular and deep, to include a wedge of perirectal fat with the specimen (Fig. 8.4). Great care should be taken

8 Advanced Surgical Techniques 65

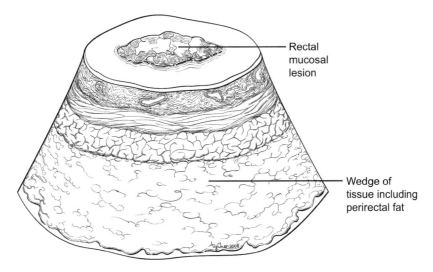

Fig. 8.4 Resection of a wedge of perirectal tissue

not to manipulate the lesion itself, grasping only the resection margin edges. Dissection continues until the extrarectal plane or the peritoneum is entered. The deep margins of the resection that are exposed are therefore the presacral plane posterior, pelvic sidewalls lateral or the vaginal wall or prostate anteriorly. Particular care is taken with anterior lesions where the prostatic or vaginal wall is in close proximity. If there is uncertainty an "on table" vaginal examination may be performed. In male patients with anterior lesions a urethral catheter should be placed to facilitate visualization of any urethral injuries. The perirectal tissue is removed in continuity with the lesion to allow accurate pathologic staging and risk stratification.

Intraperitoneal resections require particular attention. If the resection is into the mesentery a generous wedge of the mesentery is removed along with the rectosigmoid wall—being careful with larger blood vessels, which may require control or division with ultrasonic or bipolar technologies. If the resection is free into the peritoneal cavity, one must avoid injury to adjacent small bowel. Adequate relaxation must be maintained by anesthesia to prevent the bowel from herniating through the defect. Placing the patient in Trendelenberg position may also be helpful. Again, if the adjacent mesentery is visible through the rectotomy, a sample may be resected by pulling it into the rectal lumen and dividing it hemostatically. After the resection is complete, a washout of the resection bed is performed with a tumoricidal agent such as diluted Betadine solution.

Obviously after such an extended resection, particularly if the peritoneal cavity was entered, a secure closure of the excision site must be performed. Repair of the excision site is performed transversely, along the lines of a Heinike–Miculitz stricturoplasty, to avoid narrowing of the rectum. A running absorbable suture is used with silver clips in lieu of traditional laparoscopic knot-tying. To prevent misalignment two sutures are used: the first is started at the midpoint and run laterally; the second also starts at the midpoint and runs in the opposite direction. Additional mobilization of the rectum to allow for tension-free closure is sometimes required when operating below the peritoneal reflection.

Entry into the peritoneum has in the past been regarded as a complication. However closure of a full-thickness rectotomy through TEM has not been shown to be associated with increased complications. This method is a safe and commonly offered procedure even for rectal lesions above the peritoneal reflection [2].

Complications

Intraoperative complications are most commonly related to hemostasis, particularly when removing mesentery or perirectal fat. A fine monopolar grasper or bipolar forceps should be available for controlling larger bleeders. Additional injections of epinephrine solution can help to locate obscure bleeding sources. During intraperitoneal resection the adjacent small bowel is at risk of injury with the grasper or electrocautery. If this occurs, the bowel should be pulled through the rectotomy and the tear, burn or crush injury repaired with a figure-of-eight suture. If during a wide resection the vagina is entered either accidentally or intentionally to obtain margins, it should be repaired transvaginally after closing the rectal excision site via TEM. If the urethra is injured, urologic consultation should be obtained.

Postoperative leaks can be divided into immediate and delayed presentations. Leaks are rare overall, but especially occur immediately after surgery. Whether early or late, leaks commonly present with an elevated white blood cell count, fever or drainage. A water-soluble contrast enema will reveal most leaks. Extraperitoneal leaks can usually be managed with bowel rest and antibiotics, while intraperitoneal leaks may require laparotomy or laparoscopy for repair with or without pelvic drainage.

Patients are told to expect some postoperative bleeding. However, persistent bleeding on rare occasion can necessitate a return to the operating room for repeat TEM and over-sewing of the bleeding vessel. If delayed bleeding occurs in the setting of fevers and an elevated white blood cell count, it may represent a delayed leak. Most delayed leaks are treated conservatively with a course of antibiotics.

Sleeve Resection

Indications

Sleeve resection involves resection of the entire circumference of a segment of the rectum, mobilization and then reanastomosis and is indicated for circumferential polyps and rectal prolapse. A circumferential polyp is not a common finding; however, not infrequently obtaining a wide margin on a large suspicious polyp effectively leads to a circumferential resection. Patients with mucosal prolapse are particularly good candidates for a TEM approach. A resection of redundant rectal wall with creation of a high sutured anastomosis is well tolerated and more cosmetic than an open resection.

Room Preparation

For a circumferential dissection the patients are always placed in lithotomy position with lower extremities well padded. Access to the abdomen is ensured in this way, in case conversion to laparoscopy is indicated. A Foley catheter is placed on all patients. A designated MIS suite with trained MIS operating room staff is assigned to such a case as described above. The surgeon operates at the foot of the bed between the patient's legs, with the assistant at his or her side.

8 Advanced Surgical Techniques

Procedure

With the patient in lithotomy position and on a beanbag, the beveled proctoscope with a clear faceplate is first inserted to appropriately assess the depth of the lesion and to fix the TEM apparatus accordingly. Pneumorectum is then created. The proximal resection line is marked circumferentially with monopolar cautery, as is the distal resection line. Next, the submucosal and, importantly, the perirectal tissue plane is injected with diluted epinephrine to help with hemostasis. It is often helpful to tattoo a specific point on the proximal and distal resection lines to help with proper alignment during reanastomosis.

A circumferential incision is made by connecting the previously marked sites, starting with the proximal line of resection. For a polypectomy, a 1-cm margin is maintained from the edge of the polyp to account for any submucosal invasion. The rectum is then incised perpendicularly until its full thickness is divided. In order to maintain adequate caudad retraction and for alignment, four 6-in. stay sutures with affixed silver clips are placed at the four poles of the cut edge of the proximally divided rectum (Fig. 8.5). The needle of each suture is placed proximally up in the colon to be out of the operative field. These sutures can be used to provide retraction on the quadrant being operated on, without directly handling the rectum. The position of the operating proctoscope is manipulated often to improve visualization. The assistant helps position the scope, refixing the apparatus when ideal visualization is obtained. After the proximal resection line has been completed, the distal

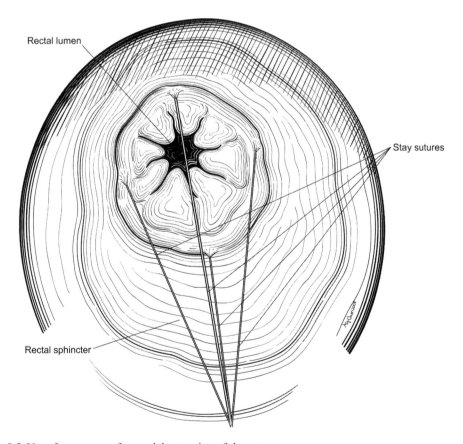

Fig. 8.5 Use of stay sutures for caudal retraction of the rectum

resection is performed similarly and the perirectal plane is dissected. For patients with prolapse, an adequate length of redundant mucosa and underlying rectum should be excised, such that the eventual suture line retracts cephalad.

The anastomosis is created using each of the preplaced absorbable sutures in a running fashion. As each quadrant is completed, the suture line is finished with another silver clip. It is absolutely essential to ensure that there is no tension on the anastomosis. As mobilization of the distal segment of the rectum is difficult, adequate cephalad mobilization is the easiest way to ensure a tension-free closure. It is equally important to prevent twisting of the anastomosis through misalignment; use of preplaced sutures and a tattooed landmark helps prevent this.

Complications

Intraoperative complications are similar to those mentioned earlier for extended full-thickness resection. A complication specific to sleeve resection is losing orientation or collapse the proximal lumen after transection. Stuffing a 4×4 sponge into the proximal colon helps avoid the later, while using the tattooing and four- quadrant suture technique helps maintain orientation.

Leaks may be divided as early or delayed leaks. All patients with a full-thickness sleeve resection are sent for a postoperative water-soluble enema on postoperative day 1. The radiologist must be cautioned about the recent repair so that a gentle, low-pressure technique is used. If disruption of the anastomosis is found on the first postoperative day, it is best to take the patient immediately for a repair. Depending on the location of the leak, the repair may be done laparoscopically or via TEM. Most intraperitoneal leaks are not subtle presentations. Patients with an immediate postoperative disruption of an intraperitoneal anastomosis will have fever, tachycardia and an elevated white blood cell count. Patients with delayed or extraperitoneal leaks may have persistent diarrhea or fevers. The workup in these patients should include a CT scan with water-soluble rectal contrast. Most delayed and extraperitoneal leaks are well managed, however, with a course of broad-spectrum antibiotics.

Postoperative bleeding is once again usually self-limited. The patient is routinely told to refrain from taking blood thinners for 5 days. Bleeding, in the setting of diarrhea, fevers and elevated white blood cell count must raise the suspicion of a leak.

Postoperative strictures are a concern following an endoluminal anastomosis, but fortunately are rare in experienced hands. Adequate mobilization of the rectum will contribute to a low stricture rate by preventing tension, but overmobilization must be avoided to preserve adequate anastomotic blood supply. Postoperative rectal strictures can usually be treated with conservative techniques (dilatation or stenting) but occasionally an operative approach is required.

Transrectal Fistula Repair

Specific Indications

TEM offers excellent visualization for effective repair of fistulae from the rectum to other midline structures; however, fistulae directly caused by neoplastic invasion of adjacent structures are not candidates for such a repair. While any fistula within 20 cm can be approached with TEM (Table 8.1), by far the most common are fistulae to the urinary tract,

8 Advanced Surgical Techniques

Table 8.1 Rectal fistulae amenable to endoluminal repair with transanal endoscopic microsurgery (*TEM*)

Fistula	Cause	Contraindication	Approach
Enterocolic	Spontaneous, foreign body, repair breakdown, infection	Opening above 20 cm, acute infection, multiple fistulae, cancer	TEM excision and repair small bowel and colon
Visiculocolic	Operative complication, infection	Opening above 20 cm, acute infection, cancer, bladder not accessible through rectotomy	TEM excision and repair bladder in layers, rectal repair and suprapubic bladder drain
Urethrorectal	Operative complication	Total disruption of urethra, cancer	TEM excision of rectal opening, mobilization of rectal/prostatic plane, urethral repair, rectotomy repair with advancement flap

usually as a result of birth trauma, bladder surgery or a rectal injury during a prostatectomy for prostate cancer.

Patient Preparation

Fistula patients are almost always complex in presentation and require special care and counseling. There are almost always several options for the repair of fistulae, such as parasacral repair, transperineal repair or a gracilis muscle advancement flap. Decisions for a minimally invasive approach for this repair should be arrived at carefully and with the full involvement of the patient and other involved specialties.

Room Preparation

High lithotomy position offers the best external access to adjacent organs (bladder, vagina, etc) but complicates the visualization of the fistula via TEM, as the lesion field will be at the upper portion of the operative field, where instrument access is difficult. We find it best in this circumstance to rotate the TEM scope 180° so that the bevel of the proctoscope faces upwards and the angled laparoscope also faces upwards, but with rotation of the camera to maintain an appropriate horizon. Alternatively the procedure may be performed with the patient in the prone position and turned supine if abdominal, perineal, vaginal or urethral access is needed. Standard room setup is otherwise used for this approach, along with the aforementioned appropriate operating room staff. Sigmoidoscopes, urethroscopes, vaginal speculums and other specialty equipment should be immediately available. A dose of preoperative antibiotic is administered. A Foley catheter is placed prior to the operation and should be placed by a urologist in the case of urinary fistulae. In cases of urethral fistula repair, the catheter will be left indwelling for 2 weeks after a successful closure to ensure healing.

Procedure

The operating proctoscope with a clear faceplate is used to locate the fistula. After the location of the fistula has been determined, the proctoscope is fixed to the bed with the

U-shaped arm and the faceplate changed to an operating faceplate. If the patient is in high lithotomy position the arm for the scope holder is placed so that it arches from above the patient's leg as the operating proctoscope is inserted upside down (bevel upwards). The initial step is isolation of the fistula. A full-thickness rectal flap is typically used for closure and may be created in a V–Y fashion or as a simple advancement flap. In either case it must be carefully marked out in advance. For the sake of this discussion, a standard advancement flap is described.

The rectal incision is initially marked using monopolar cautery. Epinephrine injections are either not used or are used very selectively (if needed for hemostasis) as perfusion of the flap is critical and is often tenuous in these circumstances. The flap is created with a U-shaped full-thickness incision on the anterior rectum distal to the fistula (Fig. 8.6). The proximal aspect of the incision is carried upward above the fistula with a wide base for the flap to ensure adequate perfusion. The flap is next elevated in a distal to proximal direction (Fig. 8.7). Midline adhesions are inevitable in the setting of a longstanding or postoperative fistula, and this can make creation of the flap challenging. After the flap has been created, the rectal portion of the fistula is isolated and excised (Fig. 8.8). All tissue removed in the case of a fistulectomy should be labeled and sent to the pathologist as occult malignancy or

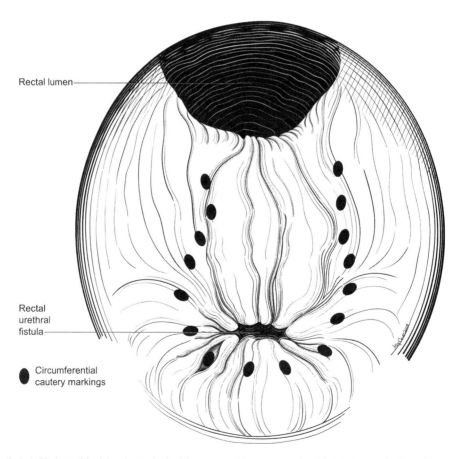

Fig. 8.6 A U-shaped incision is marked with cautery. The rectourethral fistula is seen in the midline

8 Advanced Surgical Techniques

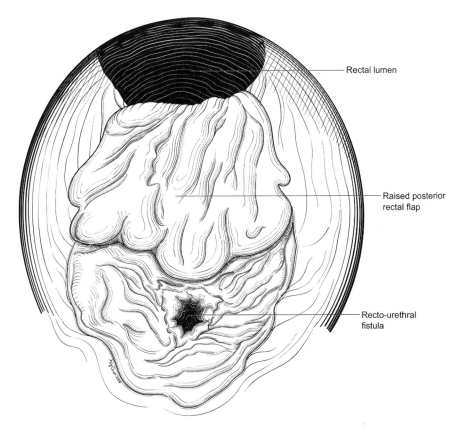

Fig. 8.7 A rectal flap is elevated to isolate the fistula tract

unsuspected Crohn's disease is always a possibility. Localization of the edges of the extrarectal portion of the fistula can be difficult. As a urethral catheter is placed preoperatively, periurethral tissue can be loosely approximated to close off these fistulae without concern for a urethral stricture. No attempt is made to close vaginal defects transrectally as they are best closed transvaginally, but bladder and enteric defects should be mobilized and brought through the rectotomy for debridement and suture repair.

With the rectum completely free of surrounding tissue and the fistula excised, additional rectal length can be easily obtained and the remaining rectal flap is now sutured into place covering the now-repaired, original defect.

Complications

As most fistulae are below the peritoneal reflection, a routine postoperative water-soluble enema need not be performed; however, if the repair was intrabdominal it is best to perform a contrast study. In addition a postoperative course of antibiotics is rarely indicated. Patients with persistent postoperative fevers or diarrhea are evaluated for a leak. Long-term failure of a TEM repair requires use of an alternative approach such as a gracilis muscle flap.

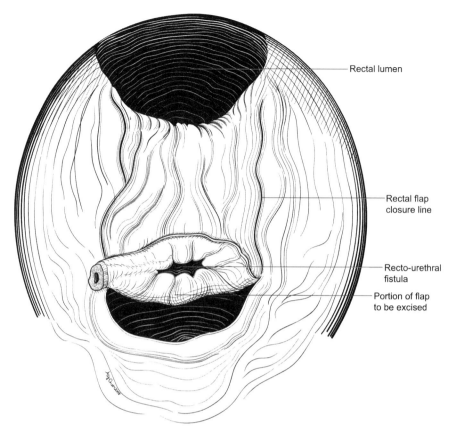

Fig. 8.8 Excision of the distal portion of the flap containing the fistula

Future Uses of TEM: NOTES

NOTES has generated considerable recent interest. This new approach to abdominal surgery involves the use of flexible endoscopes inserted by mouth, anus or vagina to exit the gastrointestinal tract and perform surgical procedures within the insufflated abdominal cavity. Early reports have described access through the stomach and several transgastric procedures have been described to date [6]. However, the transgastric approach has the disadvantage of requiring a much longer route to reach the lower peritoneum, or necessitating retroflexion to access the upper abdomen, making maneuverability of the endoscopic instruments more difficult. We have found that the rectum can be used as a safe access point to the peritoneum, utilizing the TEM proctoscope and instruments to open the rectum, maintain an access lumen and then provide a safe and secure closure after the NOTES procedure. Transrectal NOTES also offers the advantage of a much shorter entry into the peritoneum, thus allowing for more flexibility in the choice of endoscopic instruments. Indications for this approach may include partial colectomy, small-bowel resections, cholecystectomy and gynecological procedures [7]. Development of new flexible endoscopic technology makes the feasibility of such procedures all the more real. Newer operating flexible endoscopes such as the ShapeLock device (USGI Medical, San Capistrano, CA, USA) are examples of such technology [8]. The ShapeLock is an articulating flexible

Fig. 8.9 The ShapeLock device

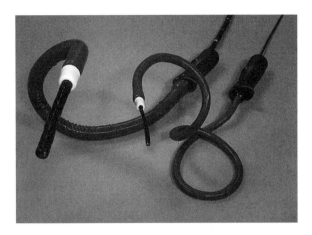

endoscopic device that can transform into a rigid metallic guide through which endoscopic instruments may be passed (Fig. 8.9). This allows the scope to be steered into position and then fixed to allow retraction of tissue and support of endoscopic instruments. This scope easily fits through the TEM scope, which also helps support it.

In a white paper published in 2005 by the Natural Orifice Surgery Consortium for Assessment and Research [9], a working group of 14 surgeons and endoscopists, one of the primary barriers to clinical application of NOTES was predicted to be access and the safe closure of the enterotomy access site. We believe that TEM offers a tried-and-tested method for safely creating and closing an access rectotomy [2]. Particularly for closure, TEM allows the use of standard laparoscopic suturing techniques rather than depending on newly developed endoscopic suturing devices, which have been designed specifically for closure of a gastrotomy site and may not be appropriate for closure of a rectotomy [10].

Conclusion

TEM has undergone a slow evolution since it was first introduced by Buess more than two decades ago. From a very narrow clinical application at its conception, TEM is today fast entering the mainstream of MIS. As more surgeons surmount the learning curve associated with TEM and become facile with its use, the indications for TEM can be expanded. With clear advantages in terms of postoperative recovery and pain, this approach provides great advantages to colorectal patients. Particularly for surgeons comfortable with laparoscopic surgery, TEM can accomplish both basic and advanced procedures and be a valued addition to their colorectal armamentarium. Finally, if NOTES should become a clinical reality, TEM may well play a role in its ultimate universal application.

References

1. Transanal endoscopic versus total mesorectal laparoscopic resections of T2-N0 low rectal cancers after neoadjuvant treatment: a prospective randomized trial with a 3 years minimum follow up period. *Surgical Endoscopy*, 19(6): 751–756, June 2005. Lezoche E., Guerrieri M., Paganini A.M., D'Ambrosio G., Baldarelli M., Lezoche G., Feliciotti and De Sanctis.

2. Full thickness intraperitoneal excision by transanal endoscopic microsurgery does not increase short term complications. *American Journal of Surgery,* 187(5): 630–634, May 2004. Gavagan J.A., Whiteford M.H., Swanstrom L.L.

3. Transanal mucosal sleeve resection for the treatment of rectal proplapse in children. *Journal of Pediatric Surgery,* 25(7): 715–8, July 1990. Chwals W.J., Brennan L.P., Weitzman J.J., Woolley M.M.

4. Long Term follow up of the Modified Delorme procedure for Rectal Prolapse. *Archives of Surgery,* 138(5): 498–503, May 2003. Watkins B.P., Landercasper J., Belzer G.E., Rechner P., Knudson R., Bintz M., Lambert P.

5. Video endoscopic transanal rectal tumor resection. *American Journal of Surgery,* 173: 383–385, 1997. Swanstrom L.L., Smiley P., Zelko J., Cagle L.

6. Experimental studies of transgastric gallbladder surgery: cholecystectomy and cholecystogastric anastomosis. *Gastrointestinal Endoscopy,* 61(4): 601–606, April 2005. Park P.O., Bergstrom M., Ikeda K., Fritscher-Ravens A., Swain P.

7. Transcolonic endoscopic abdominal exploration: a NOTES survival study in a porcine model. *Gastrointestinal Endoscopy,* 65(2): 312–318, Feb 2007. Fond D.G., Pai R.D., Thompson C.C.

8. Insertability and safety of a shape locking device for colonoscopy. *American Journal of Gastroenterology,* 100(4): 817–820, April 2005. Rex D. K., Khashab M., Raju G.S., Pasricha J., Kozarek R.

9. ASGE/SAGES working group on Natural Orifice Translumenal Endoscopic Surgery. White Paper, *Surgical Endoscopy,* 20: 329–333, 2006.

10. Endoluminal methods of gastrotomy closure in natural orifice transenteric surgery. *Surgical Innovation,* 13(1): 23–30, March 2006. Sclabas G.M., Swain P., Swanstrom L.L.

11. Laparoscopic right hemicolectomy for cancer: 11-year experience. *Rev Gasroenterol Mex,* 69(1 Suppl):65–72, Aug 2004. Franklin M.E JR, Gonzalez J.J. JR, Miter D.B., Mansur J.H., Trevino J.M., Glass J.L., Mancilla G., Abrego-Medina D.

Chapter 9
Complications

K.S. Khanduja

Transanal endoscopic microsurgery (TEM) was developed by Gerhard Buess and associates in Germany and was made available in 1983 for clinical use [1]. TEM and its instrumentation provide superior optics and excellent exposure to allow removal of favorable tumors from the rectum and the rectosigmoid colon up to 24 cm from the anal verge. It is the only one-port system in endoscopic surgery that utilizes a direct endoluminal approach to a target organ via a natural opening of the body [2]. TEM offers an alternative to conventional transanal surgery, which is limited by its use of conventional instruments and radical surgery and which is associated with a much higher complication rate.

Since its inception there has been an extensive global experience with TEM which substantiates its effectiveness and associated low morbidity rate [3–15]. TEM avoids the high complication rates associated with radical surgery, namely, anterior resection and abdominoperineal resections with the need for permanent colostomy. It avoids the frequent cardiopulmonary, genitourinary, and anal incontinence complications associated with radical transabdominal surgery [16–21]. It also avoids the high incidence of wound and fecal fistula complications associated with the Kraske transsacral [22, 23] and the York–Mason posterior [24, 25] approaches.

Morbidity and Mortality

The morbidity and mortality associated with TEM have been evaluated widely. Mentges and Buess [26] reported one mortality in a series of 522 patients. They categorized the complications as either severe or slight in 362 patients with adenomas and 126 patients with cancers; there were 34 other patients with a variety of other indications. There were 17 (4.7%) severe and 52 (14.36%) slight complications in patients with adenomas and eight (6.3%) severe and 17 (13.49%) slight complications in patients with cancers. Patients with severe complications required surgical interventions and those with slight complications did not [26]. Salm et al. [14] reported the experience with TEM in Germany that consisted of 1,900 cases from 44 hospitals, performed by 71 surgeons. There were 120 complications and a morbidity rate of 6.3%; 43 patients (2.3%) had major complications that required surgical intervention. There were three deaths (0.2%), one due to sepsis, another as a result of pulmonary embolus, and the third as a result of cardiopulmonary complications in a high-risk patient requiring a conversion to a laparotomy [14].

K.S. Khanduja (✉)
Mount Carmel Health System, The Ohio State University Medical Center, Columbus, OH, USA

P.A. Cataldo, G.F. Buess (eds.), *Transanal Endoscopic Microsurgery*,
DOI 10.1007/978-0-387-76397-2_9, © Springer Science+Business Media, LLC 2009

Smith et al. [12] reported the early experience of TEM in the USA from five surgical departments by five surgeons as "initial registry results" in 1996. There were 14 (9%) intraoperative, 23 (15%) early, and eight (5%) late complications in 153 patients. Their low complication rate in select early tumors of the rectum led them to conclude that TEM was superior to other approaches to the upper and mid rectum [12]. Steel et al. [27] reported the initial experience with 100 patients with rectal tumors from three centers in the UK in 1996. They encountered six intraoperative complications, three minor complications (two transient incontinence and one rectal stenosis requiring dilation), and one death as a result of a myocardial infarction. These early and favorable results led them to confirm the usefulness of TEM, as in the early US experience. In 2006, Guerrieri et al. [3] reported the experience of surgeons at six Italian centers using TEM to resect rectal adenomas. Of 882 patients, 588 patients were available for evaluation of long-term results. They reported that 58 (9.9%) of the 588 patients had pT1 rectal cancer on definitive histologic examination. They found only three (0.5%) intraoperative complications; 14 peritoneal entries were closed endoscopically by the TEM approach without any intraoperative or postoperative complications. Minor complications occurred in 48 patients (8.1%), major complications in seven (1.2%); the total morbidity was 11.4% with no mortality and a local recurrence rate of 4.3% after 35 months [3]. These early collective national experiences demonstrating minimal complications and highly favorable results of TEM are further substantiated by many single-institution and single- surgeon experiences [4, 7, 9, 15, 28–34].

Reports assessing the results of TEM versus those of radical or conventional transanal surgery have found it to be associated with lower complication rates and have found oncologic results comparable to those of radical surgery for favorable T1 tumors. Heintz et al. [35] in a retrospective study of 103 patients with T1 rectal cancer who underwent TEM (n = 58) versus radical surgery (n = 45) found a significantly lower morbidity of 3.4% for TEM versus 18% for radical surgery and no mortality versus 3.8% mortality for the radical operations. Langer et al. [36] in 2003 compared TEM using ultrasound or electrosurgery with conventional local and radical resections in 162 patients. They too found a significantly lower complication rate for TEM when compared with radical surgery. There was a 55.5% complication rate and a 11.1% operative intervention rate in the radical group as opposed to rates of 7.6 and 2.5%, respectively, for the TEM group [36]. Lastly, Winde et al. [28] in a prospective randomized trial compared local excision using TEM with anterior resection for the treatment of early rectal cancer. Similar local recurrence and 5-year survival rates were found for the two groups; however, a lower morbidity and significant differences in hospital stay, blood loss, operative time, and use of analgesics in favor of TEM led them to prefer TEM over anterior resection [28].

Complications

The most frequently reported complications of TEM are peritoneal entry during resection, bleeding, dehiscence, conversion to laparotomy, urinary complications, and transient anal incontinence. Others include postoperative fever, rectovaginal fistula, and rectal stenosis.

Exceedingly rare complications include postoperative cardiopulmonary complications, permanent anal incontinence or soilage, *Clostridium difficile* colitis, subcutaneous emphysema, rectovesical fistula, rectourethral fistula, small-bowel fistula, and hemorrhoidal thrombosis. Injuries secondary to positioning of the patient and postoperative hypercapnia with respiratory failure are also exceedingly rare complications of TEM.

Peritoneal Entry

Peritoneal entry during TEM can be expected during inadvertent or intentional full-thickness excision of anterior rectal tumors located more than 8 cm from the anal verge. Najarian et al. [37] reported the mean length of the anterior peritoneal reflection to be 9 cm. They did not find a difference between men and women in a study involving 50 patients undergoing a laparotomy. The ages of the female patients correlated inversely with the length of the peritoneal reflection. In the male patient it was not the age or the height but the body weight and the body mass index that correlated with the level of the anterior peritoneal reflection.

Entrance into the peritoneal cavity during resection of a rectal tumor by TEM will cause a loss of optimal distention and has been cited as a cause for a laparotomy. At laparotomy, the defect may be sutured closed after appropriate excision of the tumor [15, 32]. Other options have included a radical resection, commonly an anterior resection [5, 11, 12, 27, 38], and rarely a diverting loop colostomy [5]. The frequency of peritoneal entry appears to be between 0 and 6%. Steele et al. [27] reported six peritoneal entries in 100 patients undergoing TEM; five patients underwent transanal repair and one patient underwent an anterior resection with no further complications. Lev-Chelouche et al. [11] reported a cardiac-related death in their single case of peritoneal entry among 75 patients (the patient had severe cardiac disease and underwent anterior resection for repair of the injury).

Transanal repair and suture of the defect via TEM without laparotomy has been reported by a number of authors [3, 27, 29, 32, 38–41]. Gavagan et al. [39], in their report of 34 patients treated by a single surgeon, compared the result of peritoneal entry in 11 patients with that of 23 patients who did not have peritoneal entry. All 11 patients with peritoneal entry had endoscopic transverse closure of full-thickness defects by a single surgeon. The complications in this group were no different from those in the group that did not have peritoneal entry and there were no major complications as a result of the injury. None of the patients with peritoneal injury were treated for intra-abdominal sepsis or abscess. Guerrieri et al. [3] in their 2006 report of TEM for rectal adenomas at six Italian centers cited 16 peritoneal entries in 588 patients; two wide peritoneal entries required an anterior resection and 14 entries were repaired endoscopically without any intraoperative or postoperative complications.

Conversion to laparotomy may be needed for the repair of peritoneal entry that cannot be repaired through the resectoscope. Other reasons for conversion to laparotomy cited by Salm et al. [14] are hemorrhage, problems with suturing technique, defective instruments, patient positioning, lack of adequate visualization, and lesion size. Of 1,900 patients in the collective series of TEM patients in Germany, 50 patients (2.5%) required conversion to laparotomy. Salm et al. [14] observed an inverse relationship with the number of cases and the conversion rates; surgeons performing one to ten operations had an 11.6% rate, whereas surgeons performing more than 100 operations had a 1.2% conversion rate.

Bleeding

Intraoperative bleeding during TEM is exceedingly rare owing to the use of the monopolar high frequency needle electrocautery knife. Of 153 patients in their series, Smith et al. [12]

reported only one patient who had a massive hemorrhage during excision that required transfusion and suture ligature. Floyd and Saclarides [42] in 2006 reported the average blood loss per case decreased from 55.7 ml prior to 1996 to only 10.38 ml during the last 3 years. In contrast, postoperative bleeding is slightly more frequent and ranges from mainly minor bleeding to that requiring transfusion or surgical reintervention. Mentges and Buess [26] reported 30 patients with bleeding in a study of complications of TEM in 522 patients. Eleven required transanal ligation and 19 others did not need any intervention. In a series of 588 patients, Guerrieri et al. [3] reported rectal hemorrhage in eight patients (1.3%) that required transfusions and three other patients who required a repeat TEM suture. Stipa et al. [38] encountered six patients (7.2%) of 83 with postoperative bleeding who required a single unit blood transfusion each. Bleeding can also be controlled by endoscopic coagulation [43] or by endoscopic injection of epinephrine at the site of bleeding. Hematoma at the suture row can be managed conservatively or by perianal drainage [26].

Langer et al. [44] recommend the use of the harmonic scalpel instead of the electrocautery knife in TEM. In a retrospective comparison of the two techniques involving 63 patients, they found UltraCision[®] (UltraCision, Smithfield, RI, USA) to be associated with a lower complication rate. They concluded that secure coagulation, avoidance of thermal damage, and improved visibility resulted in reduced operative time owing to decreased bleeding and smoke. Guillem et al. [30] also preferred the harmonic scalpel when performing transmural excision for rectal cancers with TEM.

Dehiscence

Dehiscence of the site of excision in the rectal wall after sutured repair ranges from 0 to 15% [29]. In their report of 1,900 collective cases from Germany, Salm et al. [14] found 52 cases of dehiscences that were managed conservatively and four others with peritoneal involvement that required surgical attention. Lezoche et al. [45] reported eight dehiscences (three complete and five partial) among 100 patients with rectal cancers who were treated with preoperative radiation therapy and local excision using TEM. All patients were treated conservatively with intraluminal irrigation containing metronidazole and lidocaine, as well as total parenteral nutrition. Mentges and Buess [26] reported six patients who required an operation and 27 who did not in their series of 522 cases. In their series of 588 patients, Guerrieri et al. [3] reported that one patient required a repeat TEM suture and 35 others were treated conservatively using enemas containing antibiotics and analgesics and/or parenteral nutrition.

Schafer et al. [29] used proctoscopy to detect five dehiscences after TEM in 33 patients with giant rectal adenomas. Four were treated with parenteral nutrition alone and three of the four also received intravenous antibiotics. One patient required a TEM-directed repair; a recurrent dehiscence in this patient was managed by a protective ileostomy.

Conversion to Laparotomy

Conversion to laparotomy for reasons other than a complication occurs infrequently in TEM and decreases as experience is gained [14]. Salm et al. [14] reported that conversion was necessary in 50 of 1,900 cases, an incidence of 2.6%. While most authors have not reported the need for conversion to a laparotomy, few have reported the need due to lack of exposure of the entire abnormality [12, 30, 32]. Reasons cited are stenosis, angulation, narrowing of the rectum and the rectosigmoid, large bulky lesions, contour of the bony pelvis, and inability to maintain the proctoscope in the rectal lumen with carbon dioxide insufflation owing to distal location of the tumor. Smith et al. [12] in their collective series reported eight of 153 TEM cases required conversion primarily owing to lack of adequate exposure. Guillem et al. [30] encountered this in five of 32 cases, with two undergoing conventional transanal excision, while three had a low anterior resection. A thorough knowledge of the location of the tumor with preoperative proctoscopy and preferably endorectal ultrasonography when feasible may prevent the need for conversion in such cases.

Urinary

Common urinary complications include temporary retention requiring catheterization and urinary tract infection. Urosepsis and injuries resulting in rectourethral and rectovesical fistula have been reported and are extremely rare complications of TEM. Pressure on the urethra generated by the resectoscope through the anterior rectal wall is believed to cause edema and subsequent urinary retention, need for catheterization, and risk for subsequent infection. The most commonly reported urinary complications are retention requiring catheterization, with a frequency of up to 8% [31], and urinary tract infection, with a similar rate [15]. Almost all cases of urinary retention are transient and merely require temporary catheterization of the bladder [7, 9, 11, 12, 31, 40, 43]. Mentges and Buess [16] reported that 14 patients of 522 (2.68%) experienced difficulties and that six patients required suprapubic catheterization. A rectourethral fistula was reported by Lev-Chelouvhe et al. [11] after repeat TEM excision of a recurrent T3 cancer resulted in injury of the urethra. Guerrieri et al. [3] reported a patient requiring an abdominoperineal resection after TEM excision resulted in the creation of a rectovesical fistula. Stipa et al. [38] reported a single case of urosepsis among 83 patients undergoing TEM.

Anal Incontinence

Anal incontinence or dysfunction after TEM has been well documented and evaluated since the introduction of the technique. This complication is usually transient [3, 7, 11, 12, 14, 15, 26, 27, 19, 30, 32, 38, 42, 45] and rarely permanent [5, 11, 32]. Most of the dysfunction or incontinence after surgery is reported as fecal soilage or incontinence to gas, as opposed to frank fecal incontinence. Saclarides [32] reported fecal soilage in four of 73 patients, a rate of 5%, which resolved in all but one patient (1%). Guerrieri et al. [3] reported five cases of temporary fecal soiling that lasted 2 months in a series of 588 patients, a rate of 0.85%; all patients were treated with biofeedback and physiotherapy. Demartines et al. [15] reported temporary anal incontinence in six of 50 patients, a rate of 12%. This complication has been a subject of focused review in multiple reports [10, 46–52]. Kries et al. [46] and Banerjee et al. [47], reporting from the University of Tübingen in Germany, found a statistically significant lowering of the mean resting pressure but no difference in the squeeze pressure at 12 months after TEM, in 42 and 36 patients, respectively. Banerjee et al. [47] found a statistically significant loss of rectoanal inhibitory reflex in their patients postoperatively, but the anorectal function was well preserved and they stated that any symptomatic or physiologic impairment is usually transient and resolves within a year. Kries et al. [47] found no statistical difference in the frequency of bowel movements per day, continence status, and the ability to defer defecation for 5 min when comparing preoperative and postoperative status 1 year after TEM. Herman et al. [50] evaluated 33 patients using anorectal manometry (ARM), rectal barostat study (RBS), and endoanal ultrasonography (EAUS), preoperatively and at 3 and 6 months after surgery. They identified preoperative sphincter defects on EAUS, diminished resting pressure, disturbed rectoanal reflexes on preoperative ARM, and extent (more than 50%) and depth (full thickness) of resection as factors that predicted postoperative anal dysfunction. Kennedy et al. [10] added pudendal nerve study, anal mucosal sensitivity, and a continence score to ARM, EAUS, and RBS in their evaluation of 18 consecutive patients undergoing TEM. They were able to evaluate only 13 of the patients up to 6 weeks after surgery. A fall in the resting pressure without affecting continence was the only statistically significant parameter in this short-term study, and they found a correlation between operative time and a fall in resting pressure. Dafnis et al. [51] reported their findings for 48 of 58 patients obtained by a clinically validated questionnaire at a median of 22 months after TEM. Sixty-six percent of their patients reported no impact on continence and 80% reported no impact on bowel movements as a result of TEM. They did not find an improvement of the anal dysfunction over time, unlike previous studies [12, 40, 46, 47, 50]. Cataldo et al. [52] used validated functional assessment tools of fecal incontinence severity index (FISI) [53] and fecal incontinence quality of life (FIQL) [54] to evaluate functional results 6 weeks after TEM. This was a prospective evaluation using an independent research coordinator not previously involved in patient care. The numbers of bowel movements per day and preoperative and postoperative urgency were unchanged. The mean FISI scores and all four components within FIQL—namely, lifestyle, coping, depression, and embarrassment—were no different. Thus, there were no differences in continence or the quality of life as measured by validated surveys after TEM.

Rectovaginal Fistula

Rectovaginal fistula is a complication that arises after excision of tumors from the anterior wall of the rectum in female patients. A direct injury and entry to the vagina may be recognized at the time of the surgery and can be repaired directly via TEM [4]. However, fistula is often due to occult injury occurring after full-thickness excision in the area or by excessive use of electrocautery in controlling bleeding [36]. Although well described as a complication of TEM [3, 13, 14, 26, 36, 38, 43, 55], retrovaginal fistula is a relatively rare but important complication that must be avoided. Preferably, adenomas in the anterior wall should be excised by mucosectomy or partial-thickness excision. Mentges and Buess [26] reported six cases of rectovaginal fistula in 522 patients (1.15%). Four of the fistulas occurred in patients who underwent surgery for adenomas. A sliding flap was utilized to reconstruct the area in two patients, a third had a Hartmann procedure, and the fourth required oversewing of the site. The two fistulas occurring in patients operated for T2 cancers had abdominoperineal resections. Langer et al. [36] described the formation of a rectovaginal fistula 3 months after resection of a carcinoma as a result of electrocauterization to control severe bleeding; the patient then required an

Rare Complications

Fever after TEM is reported infrequently [9, 11, 12, 29, 31, 32, 42], ranging from 0 to 10.67%. Katti [31] reported eight cases with fever after surgery in 75 patients. The fever is usually transient, present in the immediate postoperative period (especially the first postoperative night), and thought to be due to transient bacteremia rather than a local site of infection [9, 33]. Persistent fever should alert the surgeon and requires a thorough investigation as to its cause. Sepsis after TEM is exceedingly rare and was reported in just two of 1,900 patients by Salm et al. [14].

Rectal stenosis has been reported [5, 12, 14, 26, 27, 38, 43] at a frequency of 0–4.3% [43], and is usually reported as a late complication of TEM. In all cases it seems to resolve after dilation or bouginage. Salm et al. [14] reported stenosis in only eight patients in their report of 1,900 cases.

Exceedingly rare complications include postoperative cardiopulmonary complications, permanent anal incontinence or soilage, *C. difficile* colitis, subcutaneous emphysema, rectovesical fistula, rectourethral fistula, small-bowel fistula, hemorrhoidal thrombosis, and injuries secondary to positioning of the patient.

Carbon dioxide gas used in the distention of the rectum can dissect through the rectal defect at the time of resection and produce subcutaneous emphysema. Transient scrotal emphysema that resolved spontaneously has been reported by Azimuddin et al [34]. Gavagan et al. [39] reported a case of pneumoscrotum in a patient who did not have any peritoneal entry after TEM. They also reported a rare case of perirectal abscess that required percutaneous drainage. Rokke et al. [4] reported a case of cervical subcutaneous emphysema, pneumoperitoneum, and pneumothorax resulting from a retroperitoneal perforation of a diverticulum during routine excision of a 1.5-cm adenoma from the proximal rectum. The injury was discovered when ventilation became difficult and subcutaneous emphysema appeared in the neck following manual insufflation of gas after equipment failure. Kerr and Mills [56] reported a case of intraoperative and postoperative hypercapnia and extensive subcutaneous emphysema during TEM that led to delayed postoperative respiratory failure requiring prolonged ventilatory support.

C. difficile colitis was reported after TEM by Smith et al. [12] and Khanduja [33]. A high index of suspicion for this complication is needed in all patients presenting with diarrhea after use of prophylactic or therapeutic antibiotics.

Positioning may lead to complications. The patient needs to be positioned in such a way that the lesion presents inferiorly on visualizing it through the resectoscope; for large lesions the patient may need repositioning during the operation. Extreme care should be exercised to prevent injuries as a result of positioning. Saclarides [32] reported a case of rib fracture as a result of positioning. This report also cited a case of hemorrhoidal thrombosis as a complication after TEM.

Cardiopulmonary complications such as pneumonia, exacerbation of chronic obstructive pulmonary disease, pulmonary embolus, myocardial infarction, and exacerbation of congestive heart failure have been reported but are exceedingly rare after TEM [5, 7, 11, 14, 15, 32].

Conclusions

TEM is clearly associated with a lower complication rate than open or laparoscopic transabdominal rectal resection; however, it has its own unique set of complications. As with any operative procedure proper preoperative preparation, and patient selection combined with meticulous operative technique will minimize morbidity and mortality. In the majority of patients, TEM is a safe, well-tolerated operation associated with minimal recovery.

As with any procedure, the surgeon should be familiar with the potential complications, their presenting symptoms, and the operative and nonoperative remedies necessary for correction.

References

1. Buess G, Hutterer F, Theiss J, Bobel M, Isselhard W, Pichlmaier H. [A system for a transanal endoscopic rectum operation]. Chirurg. 1984 Oct.; 55(10):677–80.
2. Burghardt J, Buess G. Transanal endoscopic microsurgery (TEM): a new technique and development during a time period of 20 years. Surg Technol Int. 2005;14:131–7.
3. Guerrieri M, Baldarelli M, Morino M, Trompetto M, Da Rold A, Selmi I, Allaix ME, Lezoche G, Lezoche E. Transanal endoscopic microsurgery in rectal adenomas: experience of six Italian centres. Dig Liver Dis. 2006 Mar; 38(3):202–7. Epub 2006 Feb 7.
4. Rokke O, Iversen KB, Ovrebo K, Maartmann-Moe H, Skarstein A, Halvorsen JF. Local resection of rectal tumors by transanal endoscopic microsurgery: experience with the first 70 cases. Dig Surg. 2005; 22(3):182–9; discussion 189–90. Epub 2005 Aug 13.
5. Endreseth BH, Wibe A, Svinsas M, Marvik R, Myrvold HE. Postoperative morbidity and recurrence after local excision of rectal adenomas and rectal cancer by transanal endoscopic microsurgery. Colorectal Dis. 2005 Mar; 7(2):133–7.
6. Middleton PF, Sutherland LM, Maddern GJ. Transanal endoscopic microsurgery: a systematic review. Dis Colon Rectum. 2005 Feb; 48(2):270–84.
7. Meng WC, Lau PY, Yip AW. Treatment of early rectal tumours by transanal endoscopic microsurgery in Hong Kong: prospective study. Hong Kong Med J. 2004 Aug; 10(4):239–43.
8. Ramirez JM, Aguilella V, Arribas D, Martinez M. Transanal full-thickness excision of rectal tumours: should the defect be sutured? a randomized controlled trial. Colorectal Dis. 2002 Jan; 4(1):51–55.
9. Farmer KC, Wale R, Winnett J, Cunningham I, Grossberg P, Polglase A. Transanal endoscopic microsurgery: the first 50 cases. ANZ J Surg. 2002 Dec.; 72(12):854–6.
10. Kennedy ML, Lubowski DZ, King DW. Transanal endoscopic microsurgery excision: is anorectal function compromised? Dis Colon Rectum. 2002 May; 45(5):601–4.
11. Lev-Chelouche D, Margel D, Goldman G, Rabau MJ. Transanal endoscopic microsurgery: experience with 75 rectal neoplasms. Dis Colon Rectum. 2000 May; 43(5):662–7; discussion 667–8.
12. Smith LE, Ko ST, Saclarides T, Caushaj P, Orkin BA, Khanduja KS. Transanal endoscopic microsurgery. Initial registry results. Dis Colon Rectum. 1996 Oct.; 39(10 Suppl):S79–84.
13. Said S, Stippel D. Transanal endoscopic microsurgery in large, sessile adenomas of the rectum. A 10-year experience. Surg Endosc. 1995 Oct.; 9(10):1106–12.
14. Salm R, Lampe H, Bustos A, Matern U. Experience with TEM in Germany. Endosc Surg Allied Technol. 1994 Oct.; 2(5):251–4.
15. Demartines N, von Flue MO, Harder FH. Transanal endoscopic microsurgical excision of rectal tumors: indications and results. World J Surg. 2001 July; 25(7):870–5.
16. Enker WE, Merchant N, Cohen AM, Lanouette NM, Swallow C, Guillem J, Paty P, Minsky B, Weyrauch K, Quan SH. Safety and efficacy of low anterior resection for rectal cancer: 681 consecutive cases from a specialty service. Ann Surg. 1999 Oct.; 230(4):544–52; discussion 552–4.
17. Col C, Hasdemir O, Yalcin E, Yandakci K, Tunc G, Kucukpinar T. Sexual dysfunction after curative radical resection of rectal cancer in men: the role of extended systematic lymph-node dissection. Med Sci Monit. 2006 Feb.; 12(2):CR70-4. Epub 2006 Jan 26.

9 Complications

18. Platell CF, Thompson PJ, Makin GB. Sexual health in women following pelvic surgery for rectal cancer. Br J Surg. 2004 Apr.; 91(4):465–8.
19. Nesbakken A, Nygaard K, Bull-Njaa T, Carlsen E, Eri LM. Bladder and sexual dysfunction after mesorectal excision for rectal cancer. Br J Surg. 2000 Feb.; 87(2):206–10.
20. Leveckis J, Boucher NR, Parys BT, Reed MW, Shorthouse AJ, Anderson JB. Bladder and erectile dysfunction before and after rectal surgery for cancer. Br J Urol. 1995 Dec.;76(6):752–6.
21. Maas CP, Moriya Y, Steup WH, Klein Kranenbarg E, van de Velde CJ. A prospective study on radical and nerve-preserving surgery for rectal cancer in the Netherlands. Eur J Surg Oncol. 2000 Dec.; 26(8):751–7.
22. Onaitis M, Ludwig K, Perez-Tamayo A, Gottfried M, Russell L, Shadduck P, Pappas T, Seigler HF, Tyler DS. The Kraske procedure: a critical analysis of a surgical approach for mid-rectal lesions. J Surg Oncol. 2006 Sep 1; 94(3):194–202.
23. Harvey EH, Young MR, Flanigan TL, Carlin AM, White MT, Tyburski JG, Weaver DW. Complications are increased with the need for an abdominal-assisted Kraske procedure. Am Surg. 2004 Mar.; 70(3):193–6; discussion 197.
24. Mason AY. Surgical access to the rectum – a transsphincteric exposure. Proc R Soc Med. 1970; 63 Suppl:91–4.
25. Thompson BW, Tucker WE. Transsphincteric approach to lesions of the rectum. South Med J. 1987 Jan.; 80(1):41–3.
26. Mentges B, Buess G. Complication following transanal endoscopic microsurgery. Surg Technol Int. 1998;VII:170–173.
27. Steele RJ, Hershman MJ, Mortensen NJ, Armitage NC, Scholefield JH. Transanal endoscopic microsurgery – initial experience from three centres in the United Kingdom. Br J Surg. 1996 Feb; 83(2):207–10.
28. Winde G, Nottberg H, Keller R, Schmid KW, Bunte H. Surgical cure for early rectal carcinomas (T1). Transanal endoscopic microsurgery vs. anterior resection. Dis Colon Rectum. 1996 Sept.; 39(9):969–76.
29. Schafer H, Baldus SE, Holscher AH. Giant adenomas of the rectum: complete resection by transanal endoscopic microsurgery (TEM). Int J Colorectal Dis. 2006 Sept; 21(6):533–7. Epub 2005 Aug 20.
30. Guillem JG, Chessin DB, Jeong SY, Kim W, Fogarty JM. Contemporary applications of transanal endoscopic microsurgery: technical innovations and limitations. Clin Colorectal Cancer. 2005 Nov.; 5(4):268–73.
31. Katti G. An evaluation of transanal endoscopic microsurgery for rectal adenoma and carcinoma. JSLS. 2004 Apr.–June; 8(2):123–6.
32. Saclarides TJ. Transanal endoscopic microsurgery: a single surgeon's experience. Arch Surg. 1998 June; 133(6):595–8; discussion 598–9.
33. Khanduja KS. Transanal endoscopic microsurgery. Results of the initial ten cases. Surg Endosc. 1995 Jan.; 9(1):56–60.
34. Azimuddin K, Riether RD, Stasik JJ, Rosen L, Khubchandani IT, Reed JF 3rd. Transanal endoscopic microsurgery for excision of rectal lesions: technique and initial results. Surg Laparosc Endosc Percutan Tech. 2000 Dec.; 10(6):372–8.
35. Heintz A, Morschel M, Junginger T. Comparison of results after transanal endoscopic microsurgery and radical resection for T1 carcinoma of the rectum. Surg Endosc. 1998 Sept.; 12(9):1145–48.
36. Langer C, Liersch T, Suss M, Siemer A, Markus P, Ghadimi BM, Fuzesi L, Becker H. Surgical cure for early rectal carcinoma and large adenoma: transanal endoscopic microsurgery (using ultrasound or electrosurgery) compared to conventional local and radical resection. Int J Colorectal Dis. 2003 May; 18(3):222–29. Epub 2002 Dec 14.
37. Najarian MM, Belzer GE, Cogbill TH, Mathiason MA. Determination of the peritoneal reflection using intraoperative proctoscopy. Dis Colon Rectum. 2004 Dec; 47(12):2080–85.
38. Stipa F, Lucandri G, Ferri M, Casula G, Ziparo V. Local excision of rectal cancer with transanal endoscopic microsurgery (TEM). Anticancer Res. 2004 Mar.–Apr.; 24(2C):1167–72.
39. Gavagan JA, Whiteford MH, Swanstrom LL. Full-thickness intraperitoneal excision by transanal endoscopic microsurgery does not increase short-term complications. Am J Surg. 2004 May; 187(5):630–34.
40. de Graaf EJ, Doornebosch PG, Stassen LP, Debets JM, Tetteroo GW, Hop WC. Transanal endoscopic microsurgery for rectal cancer. Eur J Cancer. 2002 May; 38(7):904–10.
41. Lee W, Lee D, Choi S, Chun H. Transanal endoscopic microsurgery and radical surgery for T1 and T2 rectal cancer. Surg Endosc. 2003 Aug.; 17(8):1283–87. Epub 2003 May 13.

42. Floyd ND, Saclarides TJ. Transanal endoscopic microsurgical resection of pT1 rectal tumors. Dis Colon Rectum. 2006 Feb;49(2):164–68.
43. Saclarides TJ, Smith L, Ko ST, Orkin B, Buess G. Transanal endoscopic microsurgery. Dis Colon Rectum. 1992 Dec.; 35(12):1183–91.
44. Langer C, Markus P, Liersch T, Fuzesi L, Becker H. UltraCision or high-frequency knife in transanal endoscopic microsurgery (TEM)? Advantages of a new procedure. Surg Endosc. 2001 May; 15(5):513–17. Epub 2001 Mar 13.
45. Lezoche E, Guerrieri M, Paganini AM, Baldarelli M, De Sanctis A, Lezoche G. Long-term results in patients with T2-3 N0 distal rectal cancer undergoing radiotherapy before transanal endoscopic microsurgery. Br J Surg. 2005 Dec.; 92(12):1546–52.
46. Kreis ME, Jehle EC, Haug V, Manncke K, Buess GF, Becker HD, Starlinger MJ. Functional results after transanal endoscopic microsurgery. Dis Colon Rectum. 1996 Oct.; 39(10):1116–21.
47. Banerjee AK, Jehle EC, Kreis ME, Schott UG, Claussen CD, Becker HD, Starlinger M, Buess GF. Prospective study of the proctographic and functional consequences of transanal endoscopic microsurgery. Br J Surg. 1996 Feb.; 83(2):211–3.
48. Wang HS, Lin JK, Yang SH, Jiang JK, Chen WS, Lin TC. Prospective study of the functional results of transanal endoscopic microsurgery. Hepatogastroenterology. 2003 Sept.–Oct.; 50(53):1376–80.
49. Hemingway D, Flett M, McKee RF, Finlay, IG. Sphincter function after transanal endoscopic microsurgical excision of rectal tumors. Br J Surg. 1996 Jan.; 83(1): 51–2.
50. Herman RM, Richter P, Walega P, Popiela T. Anorectal sphincter function and rectal barostat study in patients following transanal endoscopic microsurgery. Int J Colorectal Dis. 2001 Nov.; 16(6):370–6.
51. Dafnis G, Pahlman L, Raab Y, Gustafsson UM, Graf W. Transanal endoscopic microsurgery: clinical and functional results. Colorectal Dis. 2004 Sept.; 6(5):336–42.
52. Cataldo PA, O'Brien S, Osler T. Transanal endoscopic microsurgery: a prospective evaluation of functional results. Dis Colon Rectum. 2005 July; 48(7):1366–71.
53. Rockwood TH, Church JM, Fleshman JW, Kane RL, Mavrantonis C, Thorson AG, Wexner SD, Bliss D, Lowry AC. Patient and surgeon ranking of the severity of symptoms associated with fecal incontinence: the fecal incontinence severity index. Dis Colon Rectum. 1999 Dec.; 42(12):1525–32.
54. Rockwood TH, Church JM, Fleshman JW, Kane RL, Mavrantonis C, Thorson AG, Wexner SD, Bliss D, Lowry AC. Fecal Incontinence Quality of Life Scale: quality of life instrument for patients with fecal incontinence. Dis Colon Rectum. 2000 Jan.; 43(1):9–16; discussion 16–7.
55. Morschel M, Heintz A, Bussmann M, Junginger T. Follow-up after transanal endoscopic microsurgery or transanal excision of large benign rectal polyps. Langenbecks Arch Surg. 1998 Oct.; 383(5):320–4.
56. Kerr K, Mills GH. Intra-operative and post-operative hypercapnia leading to delayed respiratory failure associated with transanal endoscopic microsurgery under general anaesthesia. Br J Anaesth. 2001 Apr.; 86(4):586–9.

Chapter 10
Comparison with Traditional Techniques

Matthew R. Dixon and Charles O. Finne

Introduction

Transanal endoscopic microsurgery (TEM) has emerged as an alternative approach for the excision of benign and malignant lesions in the rectum. This chapter will compare TEM with traditional techniques utilized for local excision. An overview of techniques available, including conventional traditional transanal excision (TAE) as well as extraluminal excisional techniques, will be given. These will be compared with the technical approaches used in TEM as well as differences in locations of lesions that are most amenable to these approaches. Data regarding outcome following TAE and TEM for both benign and malignant lesions will be reviewed. Consideration will also be given to potential reasons for differences in outcomes with these two techniques.

Overview of TAE

TAE (after Parks [1]) has traditionally been the most widely used method for the intraluminal excision of rectal lesions. This use of this approach is limited by the location of the lesion and is best suited for more distal lesions. Lesions located higher in the rectum may be technically difficult to access. The operation may be performed in either the prone jackknife or the lithotomy position. Some have suggested, including the lead author [2], that the prone jackknife position provides better exposure. The rectum tends to fall cephalad in this position, resulting in a natural opening of the rectal lumen. This position may be further improved by strapping the buttocks apart with adhesive tape. A Lone Star retractor may improve anal eversion and allow optimal exposure to be achieved. A number of handheld retractors are available, including the Pratt bivalve retractor, the Fansler retractor and the Sawyer retractor, which may effect further exposure. Once the lesion has been identified, it is advisable to begin by marking the extent of ideal excision with electrocautery before any manipulation of the lesion occurs. An insulated electrocautery probe may minimize the damage to surrounding tissues. A goal of 1-cm margins is usually desired for most benign and malignant lesions. One method that may be used to aid in excising more proximal lesions or those that extend proximally involves the placement of stay sutures circumferentially which may then be used to prolapse the lesion distally. Care is taken to excise the lesion completely with the desired margin and avoid paring down

M.R. Dixon (✉)
Department of Surgery, Kaiser Permanente, Oakland, CA, USA

P.A. Cataldo, G.F. Buess (eds.), *Transanal Endoscopic Microsurgery*,
DOI 10.1007/978-0-387-76397-2_10, © Springer Science+Business Media, LLC 2009

toward the lesion. Depending on the histologic features of the lesion involved, either a partial thickness approach preserving underlying muscle or a full-thickness excision extending into the perirectal fat may be utilized. Once the lesion has been removed, it should be pinned out on a flat surface and correctly oriented for pathologic evaluation. Wounds may be closed with interrupted absorbable suture. This technique may also be used for lesions involving the complete rectal circumference.

Technical Differences Between TEM and TAE

TEM utilizes a binocular operating stereoscope and all of the dissection is performed under magnification. There are several significant technical differences between TEM and TAE. TEM utilizes rectal insufflation, which distends the lumen and may allow the boundary between abnormal and normal tissue to be more clearly delineated. Secondly, magnification is used for the procedure and uniform visualization and lighting are achieved. This is in contrast to TAE, where adequate visualization and lighting can be more challenging when the dissection involves the more proximal rectum. TEM does allow one to avoid forceful pulling and retracting the lesion during the dissection. This may allow surgeons using TEM to more frequently remove the specimen in one piece rather than in a piecemeal fashion, which occurs commonly with TAE. An intact specimen allows for more precise examination by the pathologist and greater confidence in securing clear margins. Lastly, TEM and TAE are often applied to lesions located in different positions. The most distal lesions, closest to the anal verge, may be easily approached with TAE but difficult to access with TEM because insufflation is lost. Lesions in the mid and upper rectum may be removed with TEM but may be impossible to access using TAE.

Endoscopic Piecemeal Excision

An additional method of local excision advocated by some for benign lesions involves utilizing a colonoscope with snare polypectomy and cautery to approach larger lesions that cannot be removed with a single pass [3]. Multiple passes may be made, allowing the lesion to be removed in a stepwise fashion. This approach may allow for safe excision of larger lesions that cannot normally be removed endoscopically, but it possesses significant inherent disadvantages. Because the lesion is removed piecemeal it is impossible to accurately describe the nature and status of the margins. This may be a reasonable technique if the lesion is pedunculated and additional tissue from the base of the pedicle is able to be sent for pathologic examination separately. However, for the majority of sessile or villous lesions this is associated with an unacceptably high recurrence rate and should be considered a method of biopsy rather than an excisional technique.

Extraluminal Techniques

Kraske

One excisional technique that has historically been employed to gain access to lesions in the mid and upper rectum while avoiding laparotomy is the posterior perineal approach to the rectum, or the Kraske approach. The surgical plan involves a longitudinal skin incision from the fifth sacral vertebrae to the external anal sphincter, allowing the coccyx to be excised [4]. The patient is approached from the right side in order to access the lower-left sacral wing. Access to the rectum is then achieved and the lesion may often be identified by palpation. A rectal incision is made longitudinally and the lesion may be excised with desired margins. Attention is taken to avoid the lesion while making the incision. Rectal closure may be performed transversely followed by closure of the levator ani muscles and drain placement.

Use of the Kraske approach has been associated with significant rates of morbidity. Wound infection, anastomotic breakdown, fistulas, hernia, stricture and incontinence are potential complications that may occur and have limited its widespread use. In addition, exposure to the proximal rectum remains limited even with this technique. Use of this approach for even early rectal cancer is controversial and the approach is considered a method of local excision rather than an alternative to radical resection because the mesorectum is not completely excised.

York–Mason

A modification of the Kraske procedure was described by Mason in 1970 [5]. This technique involves a complete division of the sphincter muscle with vertical division of the rectum. Sphincter reapproximation and repair are incorporated into the closure. Further modifications of the posterior approach have been described by other authors [6]. A recently published series originating from Duke University described 22 patients who underwent the Kraske procedure between 1992 and 1997 [7]. In this group, the authors report a rectocutaneous fistula rate of 17% and two patients required diverting stomas to allow for successful closure. The extraluminal approaches are not commonly performed today, but are included in the description of conventional techniques because they, along with open laparotomy, often represent the only options besides TEM for lesions located beyond the reach of traditional TAE.

Benign Lesions

Results of Conventional TAE

TAE and TEM have both been used in the excision of benign polyps and lesions in the rectum. Villous lesions are commonly encountered and several series have described results following excision. Preoperatively, the diagnosis of cancer cannot be completely excluded until the entire lesion can be examined histologically. Authors have reported significant discordance between initial biopsy results and final postresection pathologic findings [8]. Complete excision has been advocated as a surgical goal because benign or malignant recurrence following treatment is well known, particularly when villous tumors are involved. Using a conventional approach, several authors have described significantly high rates of local recurrence following local excision. Sakamoto et al. [9] described a series of 117 patients with large, villous adenomas and identified a recurrence rate of 30% in those who had a complete excision with the transanal technique. The reported literature is analyzed in Table 10.1. This analysis excludes patients with malignancies and attempts to

Table 10.1 Results of transanal excision (*TAE*) of benign rectal adenomas

Source	Number treated by TAE	Level (cm from verge)	Size (cm)	Recurrence after conventional TAE	Complications	Mean follow-up
Nivatvongs et al. [33]	53	7.2 (4–15)[a]	5.5 (2–12)	5/53 (9%) average time to recurrence 38 months	2 (4%) hemorrhage	31 months (3 weeks to 10 years)
Thompson [34]	24	5 (3–8)		3/20 (15%)	0	2 years
McCabe et al. [35]	14	Not stated	Not stated	6/14 (43%)	Not stated	5 years
Galandiuk et al. [36]	176	Not stated	Not stated[b]	18%: it is not clear if this rate is just those treated by TAE	20 (11%), 3 serious	5 years (0–21)
Plaja et al. [37]	14	Not stated	Not stated	2/14 (14%)	2 (14%) hemorrhage	(6–72 months)
Pollard et al. [38]	47 benign	Up to 18	Average 4–5	10/47 (22%), 5 benign and 5 malignant	5 (11%), 2 UR, 1 hemorrhage, 1 stricture requiring dilation	Mean 5.5 (0.5–18 years)
Sakamoto et al. [9]	117	6 (2–12)	3.7 (2–10)	69/117 (59%), 32 (27%) residual disease, 35 (30%) late recurrence, 2 (1.7%) recurred as cancer	10% significant requiring reoperation or transfusion	55 months (1–176)
Heimann et al. [39]	23 TAE + 23 proctotomies + 5 coloanal	Mean 4.8 (2–8)	Mean 3.0	Not stated for TAE alone 2/51 (8%) both in carcinoma in situ group	Not stated	Not stated
Keck et al. [40]	26	Mean 4.5	(5–9)	14/25 (56%), 5 persistent,9 recurrent	5/25 (20%), 1 death (colostomy closure for stricture treated by resection), 3 hemorrhage, 1 persistent incontinence	47 months (2–144)
Vargas et al. [41]	32 (25 TAE + 7 snare/ fulguration)	6 (2–15)	3.9 (1.5–9)	4/32 (12%), 2 residual disease, 2 late recurrence	2 (6%) transfusion	41 months (9–141)
Hoth et al. [42]	25?			10/26? (38%)		1.8 years
Pigot et al. [10]	198	Mean 5.6 (0–13)	Mean 5.4 (1–17)	9/193 (5%), 3 residual tumor, 6 recurrences including 2 cancers	19/198 (10%), 1 death, 4 hemorrhage (1 required surgery), 3 UR, 11 strictures (dilated)	Mean 74 months (1–168)

Table 10.1 (continued)

Source	Number treated by TAE	Level (cm from verge)	Size (cm)	Recurrence after conventional TAE	Complications	Mean follow-up
Langer et al. [43]	54	5.7 ± 2.2	2.3 ± 1.5	17/54 (31%)	9/76 (12%), 2 hemorrhage, 5 urinary, 1 venous thrombosis, 1 circulatory collapse	
Featherstone et al. [11]	50 (10 had foci of carcinoma)	5.6 (0.5–11)	Mean 5.2 (0.5–9)	1/50 (2%), 1 residual, 0 recurrences	None	Median 30 months (6–91)
Dafnis et al. [44]	71			26/71 (36%)	Not stated	Not stated
Mahmoud et al. [45]	23	6.2 ± 2.9	Tumor area 8 ± 8.8 cm^2	6/23 (26%)	2 hemorrhage (both requiring surgery)	40 months
Total 16 series	819			184/790 (23%)		

This table attempts in all series reported to exclude patients that underwent TAE for suspected benign lesions whose pathologic findings showed carcinoma. The recurrence results presented are those for the benign lesions (adenomas, dysplastic adenomas, carcinoma in situ, noninvasive carcinoma).

UR urinary retention.

[a] Includes all 72 patients, some treated by colotomy or resection.

[b] 61% of lesions larger than 4 cm occurred in the rectum. 43% of 1,440 lesions occurred in the rectum: 12% upper third, 14% middle third and 11% lower third.

look only at those who had conventional TAE with a Parks-type technique. Carcinoma in situ, noninvasive cancer, Tis, and adenomas with high-grade dysplasia are all included as benign lesions. The average recurrence rate is 23%. Pigot et al. [10] reported one of the lowest rates of recurrence, with three residual lesions and six recurrent lesions in 193 patients. They felt that a modification of the technique was responsible for their results: dissection is begun at the dentate line in the quadrant of the lesion, and a traction flap is raised vertically and used to pull the lesion to the level of the anal margin with the aim of staying in macroscopically normal tissue planes. Lesions with suspected malignancy were excised into perirectal fat. Wounds were left open to heal by secondary intention and patients were covered with systemic antibiotics for 2–5 days. Featherstone et al. [11] also reported a very low recurrence rate and believed technical details during the surgery contributed to their good results. They emphasized the avoidance of preoperative biopsies, Betadine washout to prevent implantation, completeness of excision with clear circumferential and deep margins and nonclosure of the mucosal defect to avoid needle implantation.

Results of TEM Excision

The body of literature supporting the advantages of utilizing TEM for benign lesions of the rectum is growing. TEM especially provides the ability to reach benign lesions in the middle and upper rectum which might otherwise require an extraluminal approach or laparotomy for successful excision. In 1988, Buess et al. [12] first reported the results of TEM for rectal adenomas. This series included 56 patients followed carefully. Five patients had small recurrent polyps removed by hot biopsy, and another had a flat adenoma requiring repeat TEM. The authors felt that four of these were new polyps or were undetected during the original procedure since margins were clear on the original specimens. One patient of 56 required a repeat TEM (2%). The most recent data from Buess's group is reported by Mentges et al. [13], with a mean follow-up of 2 years and a 1.7% recurrence rate (four patients of 236).

The TEM literature for benign adenomas is presented in Table 10.2 with the same inclusion criteria as for Table 10.1. The average recurrence rate for these 31 series is 5.5%, substantially less than for conventional TAE. This recurrence rate is fairly consistent within the series, though a few outliers exist. Schafer et al.'s [14] series of giant adenomas (those over 5 cm in diameter) records six patients with residual tumor (microscopic positive margins) out of 29 patients. Only four recurrences (14%) required further therapy. These results are not surprising considering the size of these specimens ranged from 5.5 cm $\times$ 2.5 cm to 13.5 cm $\times$ 5.5 cm. Suture line complications quadrupled in patients with lesions larger than 30 cm^2; one dehiscence in 16 patients with lesions less than 30 cm^2, versus four of 17 in those over 30 cm^2, one requiring a stoma.

Apart from the issue of recurrence, it certainly seems that TEM offers TAE to a group of patients not accessible to conventional methods. The majority of series of TAE have mean or median distance from the verge between 4 and 7 cm, whereas for the TEM series these values fall between 5 and 10 cm, with the occasional lesion between 18 and 22 cm. Whereas an intraperitoneal anastomosis is a rare thing in most conventional series, it occurs with regularity in most recent TEM series.

Morbidity seems comparable between the two techniques except that conversion to laparotomy is almost unheard of in the conventional group. Conversion is also rare with TEM as intraperitoneal anastomoses can be performed safely. Gavagan et al. [15] looked

Table 10.2 Results of transanal endoscopic microsurgery (*TEM*) excision of benign rectal adenomas

Source	Number treated by TEM excision	Level (cm from verge)	Size (cm)	Recurrence after TEM excision	Complications	Mean follow-up
Khanduja [46]	8	Mean 7.9 ± 1.1	3.9 ± 0.4	0/8	1 PMC, 1 fever	≥ 1 year
Said and Stippel [47]	260	Median 10 (5–22)	Mean 3.6	17/260 (7%)	10/260 (4%), 1 death (recurrent PE), 4 conversion to LAR, 1 RVF, 4 hemorrhage	38 months (3–130)
Stipa et al. [48]	15	Not stated	Not stated	0/15	5/36 (11%), 2 hemorrhages (1 Hartmann), 2 RVF, 1 stricture requiring dilation	Mean 20 months, median 22 months
Smith et al. [49]	82	Mean 7.7 ± 2.5 (3–15)	Mean 4.3 ± 2.4 (2–15)	9/82 (11%)	38/153 (25%), 14 intraoperative (9 requiring LAR), 23 minor, 1 persistent incontinence	Not stated
Steele et al. [50]	77	Mean 7.9 (1–20)	Mean 4.1 (1–14)	4/77 (5%)	3/100 (3%), 1 LAR, 1 stricture requiring dilation, 1 death (MI)	7.4 months (0–24)
Lezoche et al. [51]	40	3–12 (72%)	Not stated	2/40 (5%)	10/69 (14%), 1 PE, 2 hemorrhage, 5 dehiscence, 1 RVF, 1 stricture requiring dilation	17 months for cancers, adenomas not stated
Mentges et al. [13]	236	22% lower 1/3, 52% mid 1/3, 19% upper 1/3, 7% above 17 cm	Mean 3.8 (1–10)	4/236 (1.7%)	13/236 (6%), 1 death, 3 dehiscences requiring stomas, 3 RVF, 7 hemorrhage	2 years
Swanstrom et al. [52][a]	25	Not stated	Not stated	1/25 (4%)	3/27 (11%), 2 hemorrhage, 1 persistent incontinence	7 months (1.5–12)
Saclarides [53]	42	Mean 6 (1–12)	Mean 3.2 (1–8)	6/42 (14%)	11/73 (15%), 2 conversion to LAR, 2 hemorrhage (only 1 readmitted without transfusion), 2 *Clostridium difficile* diarrhea, 1 persistent incontinence, 1 pneumonia, 1 rib fracture (positioning), 2 minor	≥ 1 year

Table 10.2 (continued)

Source	Number treated by TEM excision	Level (cm from verge)	Size (cm)	Recurrence after TEM excision	Complications	Mean follow-up
Mörschel et al. [54]	226	26% lower 1/3, 63% mid 1/3, 11% upper 1/3	Mean 4.2, 15% larger than 6	7/163 (4%)[a]	7/238 (3%), 3 deaths (MI, PE, septicemia), 1 RVF, 5 hemorrhage	67 months (3–113)
Lev-Chelouche et al. [55]	46	Mean 7 (3–18)	Mean 2.5 (1–7)	4/43 (9%), 3 conversions to LAR/APR in adenomas not counted	16/69 (23%), 1 death after conversion to LAR, 6 fever, 3 dehiscence, 4 hemorrhage (1 transfusion), 2 persistent incontinence	36 months (5–76)
Azumuddin et al. [56]	14	Mean 8.3 (4–16)	Mean 2.8	0/14	3/14(21%), 1 respiratory failure (patient with myasthenia gravis), 2 UR	15 months
Demartines et al. [23]	36	Mean 12 cm (4–18)	Not stated	Not stated	7/50 (14%), 2 LAR (1 colostomy), 1 MI, 4 minor	31 months (11–54)
de Graaf et al. [57]	32	Mean 7.8 (0–17)	Mean area 14.7 cm^2 (estimate 3.7-cm diameter)	1/32 (3%)	13/32 (40%), 2 reoperations (bleeding and abscess), 3 UTI, 2 UR, 2 cardiac, 3 hemorrhage	Median 10 months
Nakagoe et al. [26][b]	65*	Median 5 above dentate (2–14, includes carcinomas)	2 (0.4–8, includes carcinomas)	1/65 (1.5%)	5/101 (5%), 2 conversions to LAR, 2 hemorrhage, 1 dehiscence	Median 52 months
Langer et al. [43]	57	Means 6.0 (ultrascision) and 7.7 (electrosurgery)		5/57 (9%)	6/79 (8%), 2 leaks, 2 hemorrhage, 1 RVF, 1 neurasthenia	Median 22 months (1–75)
Farmer et al. [58]	36	Mean 8.7	Mean 3.7 (1.5 × 9.8)	2/36 (6%)	5/49 (10%), 3 fever >39°C, 1 UR, 1 HBT	Not stated
Lloyd et al. [59]	68		Mean 3.4 cm	4/68 (6%)	9/102 (9%), 6 hemorrhage, 1 abscess, 1 perforation, 1 stricture	29 (3–72)
Araki et al. [60][b]	185	9.3 (4–20) based on additional 34 patients with cancer	3.9 (2.2–11) based on additional 34 patients with carcinoma	2/183 (1%)	2 immediate conversion to LAR	61 months

10 Comparison with Traditional Techniques 93

Table 10.2 (continued)

Source	Number treated by TEM excision	Level (cm from verge)	Size (cm)	Recurrence after TEM excision	Complications	Mean follow-up
Cocilovo et al. [61]	56, 1 resection, 1 resection for carcinoma, meaning 54 TEM	Mean 7.9 (5–12)	Mean 4.9 (3–8)	2/54 (4%)	2/56 (4%), 1 conversion to LAR, 1 stricture requiring dilation	Mean 39 months (9–100)
Neary et al. [62]	20	10 (5–17)	Mean 3.9 ± 2.6	1/20 (5%)	2 hemorrhage (1 transfusion)	21 months (1–48)
Tilney et al. [63]	87	7.9 (0–17)	Mean 14.7 cm^2 (estimated diameter 3.8 cm)	5/87 (6%)	5/100 (5%), 4 hemorrhage, 1 pelvic sepsis requiring diversion	Not stated
Dafnis et al. [44]	44	Median 8 (3–20), includes 14 cancers	Median 3 (1–10) includes 14 cancers	5/44 (11%)	5% immediate, 2 intraoperative, 1 conversion to LAR, 1 anal sphincter rupture (repaired), 14% long term, 2 perineal neuralgia resolved only with APR, 1 dehiscence, 3 long-term incontinence, 1 stricture	Median 22 months
Palma et al. [64]	71-1 = 70	Not stated	Not stated	4/70 (6%)	7/70 (10%) dehiscence, 3 ileostomies, 4 hemorrhage	30 months (6–54)
Platell et al. [65]	82	9.5 (4–25) all 112 patients	Mean 4.5 cm	2/82 (2.4%)	31/112 (28%), 26 UR—3 TUR prostate, 5 readmission—4 hemorrhage (2 transfusion) and 1 for pain and incontinence	1.5 ± 0.8 years
Katti [66]	58	10 (5–15)		4/58 (7%) residual, 6/58 (10%) true recurrence	2/58 (3%) hemorrhage, 6/58 fever, 4/58 UR, 1 stricture	Median 34 (24–78) months
Endreseth et al. [67]	64	Median 10 (1–18)	Median 3 (1–7.5)	8/64 (13%)	13/79 (16%), 2 conversions, 5 long-term incontinence, 5 other	Mean 24 months (1–95)

Table 10.2 (continued)

Source	Number treated by TEM excision	Level (cm from verge)	Size (cm)	Recurrence after TEM excision	Complications	Mean follow-up
Rokke et al. [68]	56	Median 5.5 (2.5–14.5)	Median 4 (0.5–11.5)	0/56	8/67 (12%), 1 conversion to LAR for unrecognized perforation, 3 hemorrhage (1 transfusion), 1 septicemia, 1 death from PE, 2 dehiscence	Median 12 months (1–33)
Suzuki et al. [69]	15	5.1 ± 2.3[c]	4.4 (4–5)[c]	0/15	None reported	2–52 months
Guillem et al. [70]	12	Not stated	Not stated	0/12 despite 2 positive margins	2/32 (6%) hemorrhage	Median 4 months (<1–18)
Guerrieri et al. [71]	530	0–>16	0–3 in 40%, 3–6 in 47%, 6–12 in 8%	23/530 (4.3%)	10 major/588 (1.7%), 1 conversion to LAR for hemorrhage, 2 conversions for wide intraperitoneal defects, 7 major complications (3 hemorrhage needing reoperation, 2 RVF, 1 leak requiring reoperation, 48 minor/588 (8%)	Median 44 months
Schafer et al. [14]	29 giant adenomas	5–15	5.6–13.5	10/29 (34%), 6 residual adenoma, 4 recurrence	5/33 (15%) suture dehiscence (1 reoperative TEM and subsequent ileostomy)	Median 36 months
Ganai et al. [72]	93	Not stated	2.9 ±1.3, 3.4±1.1 (11 in situ carcinomas)	12/93 (13%), 2 recurred as cancer	(10%), 7/136 (5%) UR, 2 hemorrhage, 2 fluid overload, 2 dehiscence, 1 abscess, 1 stricture	Median 44 months
Total 33 series	2,728			147/2,660 (5.5%)		

This table attempts in all series reported to exclude patients that underwent TEM for suspected benign lesions whose pathologic findings showed carcinoma. The recurrence results presented are those for the benign lesions (adenomas, dysplastic adenomas, carcinoma in situ, noninvasive carcinoma).

PMC pseudomembranous colitis, *PE* pulmonary embolus, *RVF* rectovaginal fistula, *LAR* laparotomy, *MI* myocardial infarction, *APR* abdominoperineal resection, *HBT* hemorrhage requiring blood transfusion, *UTI* urinary tract infection, *TUR* transurethral resection.

[a] Gasless videoendoscopic variant

[b] Variant technique, gasless TEM

[c] Includes six carcinomas

Rectal Cancer

Results of TAE

Local excision of lower rectal cancers has been an attractive alternative to radical surgery. Avoidance of the potential morbidity and mortality of a major abdominal operation (including sexual dysfunction, anastomotic leak and incontinence) as well as the possibility of a stoma provide compelling reasons for attempting to treat rectal cancers with local therapy. Some initial reviews reported low rates of recurrence following TAE of early rectal cancers. Unfortunately, the rate of local recurrence following TAE has been demonstrated in the most recently published series to be significant. One of the first studies to bring attention to this issue originated from the University of Minnesota [16]. This series included 82 patients with T1 and T2 rectal cancers treated with local excision as their sole treatment. They were retrospectively selected as ideal candidates on the basis of pathologic findings. All patients had negative margins, possessed well or moderate differentiation histologically and did not have any blood vessel or lymphatic invasion. Patients in this series were not treated with any adjuvant therapy and were followed for an average of 54 months with end points consisting of local and distant tumor recurrence, as well as survival. Of the patients with T1 tumors, 18% experienced recurrence during the study period and 37% of patients with T2 tumors experienced recurrence. Survival rates were 98% for patients with T1 tumors and 89% for T2 tumor patients.

Authors from the Memorial Sloan-Kettering Cancer Center reported similar rates of recurrence in their series published in 2002 [17]. Patients treated with local therapy alone had local recurrence rates of 17 and 28% for T1 and T2 tumors, respectively. The authors also included patients who received adjuvant radiotherapy postoperatively. Patients receiving adjuvant therapy following local excision possessed higher-risk histologic features, including a higher percentage of T2 tumors, blood vessel invasion and positive surgical margins; however, this group demonstrated similar rates of recurrence, with 17 and 24% for T1 and T2 tumors, respectively. The time to recurrence was noted to be longer in the irradiated group than in the nonirradiated group, suggesting that the addition of radiation may delay potential recurrences.

A separate series from the Cleveland Clinic published in 2005 followed 52 patients who received TAE for T1 rectal cancer [18] and were considered excellent candidates for local excision. Criteria included favorable histologic features and size less than 4 cm. Over the 55-month median follow-up recurrences were identified in 29% of patients.

Steele et al. [19] described a protocol (CALBG) involving carefully selected patients with T1 and T2 cancers treated with local excision. Patients found to have T2 tumors were then treated with adjuvant external beam radiation and 5-fluorouracil postoperatively. One hundred and ten patients ultimately met the stringent eligibility requirements, which included confirming the presence of a negative margin after excision. Patients with T1 and T2 tumors were found to have 85% overall survival and 78% failure-free survival with a mean follow-up period of 48 months.

With this background, a survey of the literature on local excision for rectal cancer by conventional techniques is presented in Table 10.3. It must be realized that these data are

Table 10.3 Results of TAE of pathologic T1 rectal cancer

Source	Number treated by TAE	Level (cm from verge)	Size (cm)	Recurrence after conventional TAE	Complications	Mean follow-up
Morson et al. [73]	91 low-risk histologic features	27% lower 1/3, 14% mid 1/3, 30% upper 1/3, 27% above	Median 2 (<1 to >5)	3/91 (3%)	Not stated	>5 years
Hager et al. [74]	39 low-risk histologic features, includes Kraske and enodoscopic excisions	Not stated	≤ 3	4/36 (11%)	1 death otherwise not stated	Median 33 months
Grigg et al. [75]	16 low to moderate risk histologic features	6 lower 1/3, 6 mid 1/3, 4 upper 1/3	< 3 cm	1/16 (6%)	None	Mean 9 years
Cuthberson and Simpson [76]	16 low to moderate risk histologic features	Mostly lower and middle 1/3	Most < 3 cm	2/16 (12%)	None significant	Mean 51 months
Gall and Hermanek [77]	36 low-risk histologic features	Not stated		3/36 (8%)	13/69 (19%), 6 requiring reoperation	Median 71 months
Gerard et al. [78]	14			2/14 (14%)		
Horn et al. [79]	17 low to moderate risk histologic features (2 endoscopic polypectomies)	9 lower 1/3, 6 mid 1/3, 2 upper 1/3	Median 2	0	Stated as low, no deaths	Median 51 months
Benoist et al. [80]	15	Not stated	Mean 3±2	2/15 (13%)	1 pelvic abscess requiring ileostomy	Mean 57 months
Coco et al. [81]	20	Mean 5 (2–8)	Mean 3±0.8	1/20 (5%)	3/36 (9%), 1 requiring colostomy	Median 68 months
Chakravarti et al. [82]	44	Not stated	Not stated	11% (estimated)	Not stated	Mean 51 months (4–162)
Steele et al. [19]	59	Not stated	Not stated	4/59 (7%)	31/110 (28%), no deaths	Median 48 months
Varma et al. [83]	24, 3 got XRT	Not stated	Not stated	1/21	Not stated	Median 6 years (0–16.6)
Blair and Ellenhorn [84]	15	Mean 4.6 ± 1.6	Mean 2.6 ± 1.1	0/15	1/20 (5%) a perforation requiring colostomy	Median 60 months

Table 10.3 (continued)

Source	Number treated by TAE	Level (cm from verge)	Size (cm)	Recurrence after conventional TAE	Complications	Mean follow-up
Balani et al. [85]	13	Not stated	Not stated	0/13	5%, no deaths	Not stated
Mellgren et al. [86]	69	5±3	2.8±1.7	18% KMP at 5years	Not stated	Mean 4.4 years
Hoth et al. [42]	10 complete	Mean 5	< 4 cm	1/10 (10%)	7%, no deaths	Mean 27 months (0–10 years)
Lamont et al. [87]	17	Median 5	Median 2.5 (1–5)	4/17 (24%)	Not stated	Median 33 months (2–102)
Paty et al. [17]	74, 7 got XRT	Median 5 (0–10)	Median 2 (0.8–8)	Actuarial local recurrence at 10 years 17%, overall recurrence 24%	Not stated	Median 6.7 years (92% followed to death or longer than 5 years)
Gao et al. [88]	36	3–8	Median 2 (0.4–3)	4/36 (11%)	5/47 (11%), 2 fistulas requiring colostomy (transsacral excisions), 2 hemorrhage, 1 stricture	Mean 53 months
Gopaul et al. [89]	32, 4 got XRT	Not stated	Median 2.7 (0.6–6)	4/32 (13%)?, 1 distant recurrence, 5/32? (16%)	Not stated	Not stated
Nascimbeni et al. [90]	70, 28 high grade, 11 with LVI	4–10	Median 2	21% 5 year KMP, 7% local recurrence		Mean 9.2 years, median 8.1 years
Madbouly et al. [18]	52	Mean 6.2 ± 2.2	Mean 2.4 (0.8–4)	15/52 (29%)	Not stated	Median 55 months
Endreseth et al. [30]	35 only 16 had R0 excisions	Mean 4.8 (2-7)	Mean 2.0 (0.2–4)	19%, 12% local, 7% distant	Not stated	(24–97months)
Bentrem et al. [91]	151, 16 got XRT	Median 6 (0–9)	Median 2.4 (0.8–5)	26/151 (17%)	Not stated	48 months (1–145)
Total	965			135/959 (14%)		

LVI lymphovascular invasion, *XRT* radiation therapy, *KMP* Kaplan–Meier estimate

from a very heterogenous group, but they do represent a broad experience in many institutions, so the results are probably representative of what can be achieved with the technique. These results may be skewed by the fact that they are more likely to include a heavier proportion of lower-third rectal cancer, which may have a worse prognosis [20].

Results of TEM

Literature supporting the use of TEM for local excision of rectal cancers is also accumulating. Mentges et al. [21] described their experience with 113 patients with rectal cancer. In this series 64 patients had T1 tumors, 33 were found to have T2 tumors and the remaining 16 patients had T3 tumors. The authors described a complication rate requiring reoperation of 7%. While eight of the 60 patients with low-risk T1 tumors elected to have further resection, 52 were followed over a median follow-up of 29 months. During this time only two patients were found to have recurrences.

Since this publication a number of series have reported excellent results when TEM is used for local excision of rectal cancer. Floyd and Saclarides [22] described 53 patients with T1 rectal cancers treated with TEM. Over a median follow-up of 2.8 years, there was a 7.5% recurrence rate. Similarly low levels of recurrence have been described in several other published series [23–26]. Lezoche et al. [27] reviewed their results with using TEM to treat patients with T1, T2 and T3 cancers and incorporated adjuvant radiotherapy in their algorithm. In their series, patients with T2 and T3 tumors who refused elective resection were recommended treatment with postoperative chemoradiotherapy. After an average follow-up period of 35 months, the authors reported no local recurrences in the T1 group and a recurrence rate of 5.4% in the patients with T2 tumors. Both of these recurrences occurred in patients who declined postoperative radiation therapy. In a subsequent publication [28], the authors reported offering preoperative chemoradiotherapy to a group of 100 patients with T2 and T3 rectal cancers and followed this with excision using TEM. During a median follow-up of 55 months, there were three (5.5%) recurrences in the T2 group and two (4.3%) recurrences in the T3 group, while two (3.8%) patients developed distant metastases.

In work originating from the University of Minnesota, we have compared recurrence rates in patients with T1 and T2 tumors treated with traditional local excision with those patients who received TEM during the same time period [29]. Patients were selected who did not receive any preoperative or postoperative adjuvant therapy and possessed clean surgical margins. During the mean follow-up period of 4.2 years, there were significantly more recurrences in the group treated with TAE than for those receiving TEM. Patients with T1 tumors displayed a 16% recurrence rate when treated with TAE versus 0% recurrence in the TEM group. In the T2 group, there were 20% recurrences in the TAE and 0% in the TEM group, though this result is skewed by the fact that all patients with T2 lesions were offered radical resection.

The published literature for T1 rectal cancer is presented in Table 10.4. These 32 series are relatively consistent in their findings. The follow-up periods are not long, but should be adequate to identify most recurrences, since patients treated with radiation, chemotherapy or both have been excluded. A 6% recurrence rate for TEM certainly suggests an advantage for TEM over conventional TAE, though TEM is less suitable for lower-third lesions. This favoring of middle- and upper-third lesions might skew TEM results since these lesions may

Table 10.4 Results of TEM excision of pathologic T1 rectal cancer

Source	Number treated by TEM excision	Level (cm from verge)	Size (cm)	Recurrence after TEM excision	Complications	Mean follow-up
Khanduja [46]	2	8 and 11[a]	1.5 and 3.8[a]	1/2 (50%)	2/10, 1 FUO, 1 PMC	>1 year[a]
Smith et al. [49]	30	8.5 ± 3.5 (3–20)	2.8 ± 1.8 (1–10)	3/30 (30%)	38/153 (25%), 14 intraoperative (9 requiring LAR), 23 minor, 1 persistent incontinence	Not stated
Steele et al. [50]	7	Mean 7.9 (1–20)	Mean 4.1 (1-14)	0/7	3/100 (3%), 1 LAR, 1 stricture requiring dilation, 1 death (MI)	7.4 months (0–24)
Lezoche et al. [27]	10, 1 got XRT	Not stated	Not stated	0/9	6/37 (16%), 1 RVF, 3 dehiscence, 2 incontinence	Mean 33 months[a]
Mentges et al. [13]	56	Not stated for the cancers	Mean 4.6 (1.2-8.9)	4/56 (7%), 2 residual in 8 resections, 2/48 (4%) by TEM alone	8/98 (8%) major, 3 dehiscence requiring colostomy, 2 APRs for RVF and phlegmon, 2 hemorrhage requiring reoperation	Mean 24 months
Winde et al. [31]	24	5 upper 1/3, 12 middle 1/3, 7 lower 1/3[a]	Not stated	1/24 (4%)	6/24 (25%), 1 hemorrhage, 1 urinary, 1 leakage, 1 compartment syndrome, 1 incontinence[a]	41 ± 25 months[a]
Heintz et al. [92]	44 low risk	10 upper 1/3, 16 middle 1/3, 20 lower 1/3[a]	2.5 ± 1.5[a]	0/44	1/44 (2%), 1 RVF	52 ± 23 months[a]
Heintz et al. [92]	12 high risk	1 upper 1/3, 4 middle 1/3, 7 lower 1/3[a]	3.5 ± 1.8[a]	4/12 (33%), 3 cancer deaths	1/12 (8%), 1 dehiscence	43 ± 22 months[a]
Lev-Chelouche et al. [55]	10, 2 conversion to LAR	Mean 8 (3–15) includes all cancers	Mean 3 (2–5), includes all cancers	0/8	16/69 (23%), 1 death after conversion to LAR, 6 fever, 3 dehiscence, 4 hemorrhage (1 transfusion), 2 persistent incontinence	33 months (4–72)
Azumuddin et al. [56]	9	Mean 8.3 (4–16)	Mean 2.8	0/9	6/31 (19%)	14 ± 6 months
Demartines et al. [23]	9, 1 had adjuvant therapy, 1 resection	Not stated	Not stated	1/8 (13%)	7/50 (14%), 2 laparotomies (1 colostomy), 1 MI, 4 minor	30.6 (11–54)

Table 10.4 (continued)

Source	Number treated by TEM excision	Level (cm from verge)	Size (cm)	Recurrence after TEM excision	Complications	Mean follow-up
de Graaf et al. [57]	21	Median 8 (0–17)	Mean 3.8	2/19 (11%)	13/32 (40%), 2 reoperations (bleeding and abscess), 3 UTI, 2 UR, 2 cardiac, 3 hemorrhage	Mean 12.5 months, median 7 months (1–47)
Nakagoe et al. [26][b]	23, 8 resections, meaning 15 TEM only	Median 5 (2–14)	Median 2 (0.4–8)	0/15	5/101 (5%), 2 conversions to LAR, 2 hemorrhage, 1 dehiscence	Median 52 months (12–91)
Langer et al. [93]	17	Median 6.9 ± 2.8	Mean 3.4 ± 1.5	3/17 (18%)	2/17 (12%)	23 ± 17 months
Lloyd et al. [59]	6	3.5–9	Mean 2.6 (1–3.4)[a]	1/6 (17%), 1 residual got resected	9/102 (9%), 6 hemorrhage, 1 abscess, 1 perforation, 1 stricture	Mean 28 months (12–47)[a]
Araki et al. [60][c]	22	Mean 9.3 (4–20)	Mean 3.9 (2.2–11)	0/22	20/217 (9%), 1 death, 2 immediate conversion to LAR, 12 soiling, 5 fever, 2 hemorrhage	61 months
Lee et al. [94]	52	Mean 6.7 ± 3.2	Mean 2.3 ± 0.9	4% KMP	3/74 (4%), 1 hemorrhage, 1 incontinence, 1 urinary	Mean 31 months
Neary et al. [62]	5	Mean 10 (5–17)	Mean 3.9 ± 2.6	0/5	6/19 (32%), 1 UR, 5 hemorrhage	20 months (1–47)
Tilney et al. [63]	8-4 resections = 4	Mean 7.9 (0–17)	Mean 3.8	0/4	5/100 (5%), 4 hemorrhage, 1 diversion for sepsis	Not stated
Dafnis et al. [44]	10	Median 8 (3–20)	Median (1–10)	1/10 (10%)	5% immediate, 2 intraoperative, 1 conversion to LAR, 1 anal sphincter rupture (repaired), 14% long term, 2 perineal neuralgia resolved only with APR, 1 dehiscence, 3 long-term incontinence, 1 stricture	Median 22 months
Palma et al. [64]	21-3 immediate resections = 18 (2 had chemoXRT)	Mean 9.4 ± 2.3		1/18 (6%)	None in the T1 cases	30 months (6–54)

Table 10.4 (continued)

Source	Number treated by TEM excision	Level (cm from verge)	Size (cm)	Recurrence after TEM excision	Complications	Mean follow-up
Katti [66]	9	Not stated	Not stated	1/9 (11%)	4/17 (24%), 2 fever, 2 catheterized	Mean 36 months (25–76)
Duek et al. [24]	25	≤ 10 cm	≤ 3 cm	0/25	None 0/25	Mean 4.3 years[a]
Endreseth et al. [30]	8	Median 10	Median 3	0/8	Not stated for malignant lesions	Mean 24 months(1–95)
Floyd and Saclarides [22]	53	Mean 7 (0–13)[a]	Mean 2.4 (1–10)	4/53 (7.5%)	10/53 (19%), 3 hemorrhage, 2 transient incontinence, 3 tenesmus, 2 UTI	Mean 2.8 years[a]
Rokke et al. [68]	6, 2 resections	Not stated	Not stated	0/4	8/67 (12%), 1 conversion to LAR for unrecognized perforation, 3 hemorrhage (1 transfusion), 1 septicemia, 1 death from PE, 2 dehiscence	Median 12 months (1–33)
Susuki et al. [69]	6, 2 resections	Not stated	Not stated	1/4 (25%)	None	Mean 27 months (2–52)
Guillem et al. [70]	9	Median 9 (3–15)	Not stated	0/9	3/32, 2 hemorrhage, 1 seepage for 1 year	Median 16 weeks (0.1–72 weeks)
Guerrieri et al. [71]	58	Not stated	Not stated	0/58	10 major/588 (1.7%), 1 conversion to laparotomy for hemorrhage, 2 conversions for wide intraperitoneal defects, 7 major complications (3 hemorrhage needing reoperation, 2 RVF, 1 leak requiring reoperation, 48 minor/ 588 (8%)	Median 35 months[a]
Schafer et al. [14]	4, 2 resections	Not stated	Not stated	0/2	5/33 (15%) suture dehiscence (1 reoperative TEM and subsequent ileostomy)	4.7 (2.1–7.5) years

				Table 10.4 (continued)		
Source	Number treated by TEM excision	Level (cm from verge)	Size (cm)	Recurrence after TEM excision	Complications	Mean follow-up
Ganai et al. [72]	21, 1 had chemoXRT	Not stated	Mean 3.3 ± 1.2[a]	2/21 (9.5%) + 2 as benign adenomas	(10% of 136), 7 UR, 2 hemorrhage, 2 fluid overload, 2 dehiscence, 1 abscess, 1 stricture	Mean 43 ± 31 months[a]
Stipa et al. [95]	23, 4 with XRT	Mean 6.8 (1–13)	Mean 2.9 (0.3–8)	2/19 (11%)	12/69 (17%), 6 perforation (4 laparotomies), 2 hemorrhage, 1 RVF, 1 minor incontinence, 1 UTI, 1 DVT	Median 6.5 years (5–10.5)
Maslekar et al. [96]	27	Median 9 (4–11)[a]		0/27		Median 40 months[a]
Total 33 series	618			34/616 (5.5%)		

FUO fever of undertmined origin, *DVT* deep vein thrombosis
[a] Applies only to the lesions listed
[b] Gasless video technique
[c] Gasless TEM

10 Comparison with Traditional Techniques

have a better outcome [20]. Certainly, these combined results support the use of TEM excision (over TAE) for T1 rectal cancer.

Comparison Studies

Endreseth et al. [30] compared conventional TAE with radical resection of T1 rectal cancer in a retrospective analysis of the Norwegian National Rectal Cancer Project, a prospectively collected database. Selection of the procedure was done by local surgeons without regard to any set of guidelines. Thirty-five patients underwent TAE compared with 256 resections, but only 16 of the 35 had R0 excisions. Twelve percent of the TAE group had local recurrences without any distant metastasis, whereas 6% of the resection group had local recurrences, with another 7% developing metastatic disease at 5-year follow-up. The disease-free 5-year survival rate was 64% (local excision) and 77% (resection). Only one of the failures in the TAE group underwent salvage, thought to be related to poor operative risk in this group. Postoperative mortality was similar in the two groups, 2.9% (TAE) and 2.3% (resection). In the resection group, 34% had permanent stomas and 18% temporary diversion.

TEM has been compared with resection in four studies (Table 10.5). Winde et al. [31]reported the only randomized controlled trial, but for these selected patients it would appear that for T1 lesions the end result for TEM and resection is similar, resection carrying

Table 10.5 Direct comparison of TEM and resection

	TEM		Resection	
	T1	T2	T1	T2
Lee et al. [94] (2003)				
Number				
Recurrence (%)	51	22	17	83
Disease-free survival (%)	4	19	0	9.4
	96	80	94	83
Mean distance from verge (cm)	6.7 ± 3.2		7.5 ± 4	
Mean size (cm)	2.3 ±0.95		3.78 ± 1.5	
Complications (%)	4		48	
Heintz et al. [92]				
Number	46 low risk		34 low risk	
Recurrence	2 (4%)		2 (6%)	
5-year survival (%)	79		81	
Tumor size (cm)	2.5 ± 1.5		2.9 ± 1.6	
Complications	1 (2%)		5 (15%), 2 deaths	
Langer et al. [43]				
Number	20		18	
Recurrence	2 (10%)		None	
2-year survival (%)	100		96	
Complications	6 (30%)		15 (56%), 1 death	
Winde et al. [31]				
Number	24		26	
Recurrence	2?[a] (8%)		1 (4%) distant	
5-year survival (%)	96%		96%	

[a]One local recurrence. A second patient died of unknown cause without autopsy and was presumed to have recurrence.

greater risk of serious complication and therefore evening the score with TEM's greater risk of recurrence. The need for larger controlled trials is evident.

Middleton et al. [32] provided an exhaustive review of TEM and came to the conclusion: "...transanal endoscopic microsurgery does appear to result in fewer recurrences than those with direct local excision in adenomas and thus may be a useful procedure for several small niches of patient types—i.e. for large benign lesions of the middle to upper third of the rectum, for T1 low-risk rectal cancers...."

Discussion

TAE has proven to be a useful technique for the excision of rectal lesions and is able to provide access to lesions that may be difficult to remove using standard local excision. Results following TEM, particularly considering rates of local recurrence, have been generally positive and in many cases appear to surpass the results using local techniques. There are several possibilities for these differences in results when both benign and malignant lesions are considered.

As stated previously, there are significant technical differences between TEM and any of the conventional approaches. For one, TEM allows the excision to be performed using magnification, which may allow a more precise determination of the boundary between normal and abnormal tissue. The use of rectal insufflation also distends the rectal lumen further, improving the visibility. These technical differences may explain some of the differences reported when excising benign lesions. While low recurrence rates using traditional techniques excising benign villous tumors have been reported and appear to possible with modified technique [10], TEM appears to be associated with a decrease in recurrence rate. Part of this may be related to the fact that the technique of TEM promotes removing the specimen in one piece and allowing for careful histologic study of the margins. TEM is technically challenging and there certainly may be a selection bias in that surgeons who have been drawn to TEM and enjoy this technique may be a bit more precise and deliberate than the group of surgeons using conventional techniques.

When malignant lesions are considered, it is important to remember that the lesions removed with TEM and TAE are located in different areas of the rectum. The lowest-lying lesions may be impossible to approach with TEM and are excised locally. Some authors have reported that the level from the anal verge may be an important risk factor for predicting local recurrence of early rectal cancers as distal tumors may be more likely to harbor occult nodal metastases [20]. This may represent an inherent selection bias that should be considered when interpreting these results and may account for some of the observed differences. Despite this difference, many nonrandomized series have demonstrated differences in recurrence rates between the techniques.

TEM is of definite value in excising benign lesions in the upper and middle rectum which would otherwise require a more radical approach using laparotomy and should be considered the preferred approach in this patient group. TEM appears to offer favorable outcomes when used for local excision of other lesions as well. When local excision is to be used as primary therapy for T2 tumors, the use of radiotherapy and whether it is given preoperatively or postoperatively is currently being addressed in ongoing clinical trials. In either case, TEM may be safely incorporated as the excisional method for lesions amenable to this technique.

10 Comparison with Traditional Techniques

At this point, TEM has demonstrated that it plays an important role in local excision. In the studies previously published, results appear to be favorable with this technique. Additional data and experience with a wider range of surgeons will likely elucidate and quantify the nature of the benefit and the exact benefit that TEM provides.

References

1. Parks AG. A technique for excising extensive villous papillomatous change in the lower rectum. *Proc R Soc Med* 1968;61(5):441–2.
2. Finne CO. Transanal excision of benign lesions of the anorectum. *Operative Techniques in General Surg* 2001;3:183–199.
3. Kume K, Murata I, Yoshikawa I, Yamasaki M, Kanda K, Otsuki M. Endoscopic piecemeal mucosal resection of large colorectal tumors. *Hepatogastroenterology* 2005;52(62):429–32.
4. Wilson SE, Gordon HE. Excision of rectal lesions by the Kraske approach. *Am J Surg* 1969;118(2):213–7.
5. Mason AY. Surgical access to the rectum–a transsphincteric exposure. *Proc R Soc Med* 1970;63 Suppl:91–4.
6. Sweeney WB, Deshmukh N. Modified Kraske approach for disease of the mid-rectum. *Am J Gastroenterol* 1991;86(1):75–8.
7. Onaitis M, Ludwig K, Perez-Tamayo A, Gottfried M, Russell L, Shadduck P, et al. The Kraske procedure: a critical analysis of a surgical approach for mid-rectal lesions. *J Surg Oncol* 2006;94(3):194–202.
8. Taylor EW, Thompson H, Oates GD, Dorricott NJ, Alexander-Williams J, Keighley MR. Limitations of biopsy in preoperative assessment of villous papilloma. *Dis Colon Rectum* 1981;24(4):259–62.
9. Sakamoto GD, MacKeigan JM, Senagore AJ. Transanal excision of large, rectal villous adenomas. *Dis Colon Rectum* 1991;34(10):880–5.
10. Pigot F, Bouchard D, Mortaji M, Castinel A, Juguet F, Chaume JC, et al. Local excision of large rectal villous adenomas: long-term results. *Dis Colon Rectum* 2003;46(10):1345–50.
11. Featherstone JM, Grabham JA, Fozard JB. Per-anal excision of large, rectal, villous adenomas. *Dis Colon Rectum* 2004;47(1):86–9.
12. Buess G, Kipfmuller K, Ibald R, Heintz A, Hack D, Braunstein S, et al. Clinical results of transanal endoscopic microsurgery. *Surg Endosc* 1988;2(4):245–50.
13. Mentges B, Buess G, Schafer D, Manncke K, Becker HD. Local therapy of rectal tumors. *Dis Colon Rectum* 1996;39(8):886–92.
14. Schafer H, Baldus SE, Holscher AH. Giant adenomas of the rectum: complete resection by transanal endoscopic microsurgery (TEM). *Int J Colorectal Dis* 2006;21(6):533–7.
15. Gavagan JA, Whiteford MH, Swanstrom LL. Full-thickness intraperitoneal excision by transanal endoscopic microsurgery does not increase short-term complications. *Am J Surg* 2004;187(5):630–4.
16. Garcia-Aguilar J, Mellgren A, Sirivongs P, Buie D, Madoff RD, Rothenberger DA. Local excision of rectal cancer without adjuvant therapy: a word of caution. *Ann Surg* 2000;231(3):345–51.
17. Paty PB, Nash GM, Baron P, Zakowski M, Minsky BD, Blumberg D, et al. Long-term results of local excision for rectal cancer. *Ann Surg* 2002;236(4):522–29; discussion 529–30.
18. Madbouly KM, Remzi FH, Erkek BA, Senagore AJ, Baeslach CM, Khandwala F, et al. Recurrence after transanal excision of T1 rectal cancer: should we be concerned? *Dis Colon Rectum* 2005;48(4):711–9; discussion 719–21.
19. Steele GD, Jr., Herndon JE, Bleday R, Russell A, Benson A, 3rd, Hussain M, et al. Sphincter-sparing treatment for distal rectal adenocarcinoma. *Ann Surg Oncol* 1999;6(5):433–41.
20. Nascimbeni R, Burgart LJ, Nivatvongs S, Larson DR. Risk of lymph node metastasis in T1 carcinoma of the colon and rectum. *Dis Colon Rectum* 2002;45(2):200–6.
21. Mentges B, Buess G, Effinger G, Manncke K, Becker HD. Indications and results of local treatment of rectal cancer. *Br J Surg* 1997;84(3):348–51.
22. Floyd ND, Saclarides TJ. Transanal endoscopic microsurgical resection of pT1 rectal tumors. *Dis Colon Rectum* 2006;49(2):164–8.
23. Demartines N, von Flue MO, Harder FH. Transanal endoscopic microsurgical excision of rectal tumors: indications and results. *World J Surg* 2001;25(7):870–5.

24. Duek SD, Krausz MM, Hershko DD. Transanal endoscopic microsurgery for rectal cancer. *Isr Med Assoc J* 2005;7(7):435–8.
25. Marks JH, Marchionni C, Marks GJ. Transanal endoscopic microsurgery in the treatment of select rectal cancers or tumors suspicious for cancer. *Surg Endosc* 2003;17(7):1114–7.
26. Nakagoe T, Ishikawa H, Sawai T, Tsuji T, Tanaka K, Ayabe H. Surgical technique and outcome of gasless video endoscopic transanal rectal tumour excision. *Br J Surg* 2002;89(6):769 74.
27. Lezoche E, Guerrieri M, Paganini AM, Feliciotti F. Transanal endoscopic microsurgical excision of irradiated and nonirradiated rectal cancer. A 5-year experience. *Surg Laparosc Endosc* 1998;8(4):249–56.
28. Lezoche E, Guerrieri M, Paganini AM, Baldarelli M, De Sanctis A, Lezoche G. Long-term results in patients with T2-3 N0 distal rectal cancer undergoing radiotherapy before transanal endoscopic microsurgery. *Br J Surg* 2005;92(12):1546–52.
29. Dixon M, Finne C, Madoff R, Goldberg J, Mellgren A, Alavi K. Transanal endoscopic microsurgery improves outcome in local treatment of early rectal cancer. In: American Society of Colon and Rectal Surgeons Annual Scientific Meeting. Seattle, WA; 2006.
30. Endreseth BH, Myrvold HE, Romundstad P, Hestvik UE, Bjerkeset T, Wibe A. Transanal excision vs. major surgery for T1 rectal cancer. *Dis Colon Rectum* 2005;48(7):1380–8.
31. Winde G, Nottberg H, Keller R, Schmid KW, Bunte H. Surgical cure for early rectal carcinomas (T1). Transanal endoscopic microsurgery vs. anterior resection. *Dis Colon Rectum* 1996;39(9):969–76.
32. Middleton PF, Sutherland LM, Maddern GJ. Transanal endoscopic microsurgery: a systematic review. *Dis Colon Rectum* 2005;48(2):270–84.
33. Nivatvongs S, Balcos EG, Schottler JL, Goldberg SM. Surgical management of large villous tumors of the rectum. *Dis Colon Rectum* 1973;16(6):508–14.
34. Thompson JP. Treatment of Sessile Villous and Tubulovillous Adenomas of the Rectum: Experience of St. Msrk's Hospital, 1963–1972. *Dis Colon Rectum* 1977;20(6):467–472.
35. McCabe JC, McSherry CK, Sussman EB, Gray GF. Villous tumors of the large bowel. *Am J Surg* 1973;126(3):336–42.
36. Galandiuk S, Fazio VW, Jagelman DG, Lavery IC, Weakley FA, Petras RE, et al. Villous and tubulovillous adenomas of the colon and rectum. A retrospective review, 1964–1985. *Am J Surg* 1987;153(1):41–7.
37. Plaja S, La Rosa C, Sparacino G, Russo A, Modica G, Bazan P. Management of villous adenomas of the rectum. *Colo-proctology* 1987;9(5):277–280.
38. Pollard SG, Macfarlane R, Everett WG. Villous tumours of the large bowel. *Br J Surg* 1988;75(9):910–2.
39. Heimann TM, Oh C, Steinhagen RM, Greenstein AJ, Perez C, Aufses AH, Jr. Surgical treatment of tumors of the distal rectum with sphincter preservation. *Ann Surg* 1992;216(4):432–6; discussion 436–7.
40. Keck JO, Schoetz DJ, Jr., Roberts PL, Murray JJ, Coller JA, Veidenheimer MC. Rectal mucosectomy in the treatment of giant rectal villous tumors. *Dis Colon Rectum* 1995;38(3):233–8.
41. Vargas HD, Beck DE, Opelka FG, Hicks TC, Timmcke AE, Gathright JB. Recurrence of Rectal Villous Adenoma Following Transanal Excision. *Perspectives in Colon and Rectal Surgery* 2000;13(2):7–15.
42. Hoth JJ, Waters GS, Pennell TC. Results of local excision of benign and malignant rectal lesions. *Am Surg* 2000;66(12):1099–103.
43. Langer C, Liersch T, Suss M, Siemer A, Markus P, Ghadimi BM, et al. Surgical cure for early rectal carcinoma and large adenoma: transanal endoscopic microsurgery (using ultrasound or electrosurgery) compared to conventional local and radical resection. *Int J Colorectal Dis* 2003;18(3):222–9.
44. Dafnis G, Pahlman L, Raab Y, Gustafsson UM, Graf W. Transanal endoscopic microsurgery: clinical and functional results. *Colorectal Dis* 2004;6(5):336–42.
45. Mahmoud N, Madoff RD, Rothenberger DA, Finne CO. TEM reduces the incidence of positive margins compared with transanal excision for rectal tumors. In: American Society of Colon and Rectal Surgeons Annual Meeting Poster Session. San Diego, California; 2001.
46. Khanduja KS. Transanal endoscopic microsurgery. Results of the initial ten cases. *Surg Endosc* 1995;9(1):56–60.
47. Said S, Stippel D. Transanal endoscopic microsurgery in large, sessile adenomas of the rectum. A 10-year experience. *Surg Endosc* 1995;9(10):1106–12.
48. Stipa S, Lucandri G, Stipa F, Chiavellati L, Sapienza P. Local excision of rectal tumours with transanal endoscopic microsurgery. *Tumori* 1995;81(3 Suppl):50–6.

10 Comparison with Traditional Techniques

49. Smith LE, Ko ST, Saclarides T, Caushaj P, Orkin BA, Khanduja KS. Transanal endoscopic microsurgery. Initial registry results. *Dis Colon Rectum* 1996;39(10 Suppl):S79–84.
50. Steele RJ, Hershman MJ, Mortensen NJ, Armitage NC, Scholefield JH. Transanal endoscopic microsurgery – initial experience from three centres in the United Kingdom. *Br J Surg* 1996;83(2):207–10.
51. Lezoche E, Guerrieri M, Paganini A, Feliciotti F, Di Pietrantonj F. Is transanal endoscopic microsurgery (TEM) a valid treatment for rectal tumors? *Surg Endosc* 1996;10(7):736–41.
52. Swanstrom LL, Smiley P, Zelko J, Cagle L. Video endoscopic transanal-rectal tumor excision. *Am J Surg* 1997;173(5):383–5.
53. Saclarides TJ. Transanal endoscopic microsurgery: a single surgeon's experience. *Arch Surg* 1998;133(6):595–8; discussion 598–9.
54. Morschel M, Heintz A, Bussmann M, Junginger T. Follow-up after transanal endoscopic microsurgery or transanal excision of large benign rectal polyps. Langenbecks *Arch Surg* 1998;383(5):320–4.
55. Lev-Chelouche D, Margel D, Goldman G, Rabau MJ. Transanal endoscopic microsurgery: experience with 75 rectal neoplasms. *Dis Colon Rectum* 2000;43(5):662–7; discussion 667–8.
56. Azimuddin K, Riether RD, Stasik JJ, Rosen L, Khubchandani IT, Reed JF, 3rd. Transanal endoscopic microsurgery for excision of rectal lesions: technique and initial results. *Surg Laparosc Endosc Percutan Tech* 2000;10(6):372–8.
57. de Graaf EJ, Doornebosch PG, Stassen LP, Debets JM, Tetteroo GW, Hop WC. Transanal endoscopic microsurgery for rectal cancer. *Eur J Cancer* 2002;38(7):904–10.
58. Farmer KC, Wale R, Winnett J, Cunningham I, Grossberg P, Polglase A. Transanal endoscopic microsurgery: the first 50 cases. *ANZ J Surg* 2002;72(12):854–6.
59. Lloyd GM, Sutton CD, Marshall LJ, Baragwanath P, Jameson JS, Scott AD. Transanal endoscopic microsurgery–lessons from a single UK centre series. *Colorectal Dis* 2002;4(6):467–72.
60. Araki Y, Isomoto H, Shirouzu K. Video-assisted gasless transanal endoscopic microsurgery: a review of 217 cases of rectal tumors over the past 10 years. *Dig Surg* 2003;20(1):48–52.
61. Cocilovo C, Smith LE, Stahl T, Douglas J. Transanal endoscopic excision of rectal adenomas. *Surg Endosc* 2003;17(9):1461–3.
62. Neary P, Makin GB, White TJ, White E, Hartley J, MacDonald A, et al. Transanal endoscopic microsurgery: a viable operative alternative in selected patients with rectal lesions. *Ann Surg Oncol* 2003;10(9):1106–11.
63. Tilney HS, Heriot AG, Pearson T, Simson JNL. Transanal endoscopic microsurgery: one hundred consecutive cases. *British J Surg* 2003;90(Suppl. 1):67.
64. Palma P, Freudenberg S, Samel S, Post S. Transanal endoscopic microsurgery: indications and results after 100 cases. *Colorectal Dis* 2004;6(5):350–5.
65. Platell C, Denholm E, Makin G. Efficacy of transanal endoscopic microsurgery in the management of rectal polyps. *J Gastroenterol Hepatol* 2004;19(7):767–72.
66. Katti G. An evaluation of transanal endoscopic microsurgery for rectal adenoma and carcinoma. *Jsls* 2004;8(2):123–6.
67. Endreseth BH, Wibe A, Svinsas M, Marvik R, Myrvold HE. Postoperative morbidity and recurrence after local excision of rectal adenomas and rectal cancer by transanal endoscopic microsurgery. *Colorectal Dis* 2005;7(2):133–7.
68. Rokke O, Iversen KB, Ovrebo K, Maartmann-Moe H, Skarstein A, Halvorsen JF. Local resection of rectal tumors by transanal endoscopic microsurgery: experience with the first 70 cases. *Dig Surg* 2005;22(3):182–9; discussion 189–90.
69. Suzuki H, Furukawa K, Kan H, Tsuruta H, Matsumoto S, Akiya Y, et al. The role of transanal endoscopic microsurgery for rectal tumors. *J Nippon Med Sch* 2005;72(5):278–84.
70. Guillem JG, Chessin DB, Jeong SY, Kim W, Fogarty JM. Contemporary applications of transanal endoscopic microsurgery: technical innovations and limitations. *Clin Colorectal Cancer* 2005;5(4):268–73.
71. Guerrieri M, Baldarelli M, Morino M, Trompetto M, Da Rold A, Selmi I, et al. Transanal endoscopic microsurgery in rectal adenomas: experience of six Italian centres. *Dig Liver Dis* 2006;38(3):202–7.
72. Ganai S, Kanumuri P, Rao RS, Alexander AI. Local recurrence after transanal endoscopic microsurgery for rectal polyps and early cancers. *Ann Surg Oncol* 2006;13(4):547–56.
73. Morson BC, Bussey HJ, Samoorian S. Policy of local excision for early cancer of the colorectum. *Gut* 1977;18(12):1045–50.
74. Hager T, Gall FP, Hermanek P. Local excision of cancer of the rectum. *Dis Colon Rectum* 1983;26(3):149–51.

75. Grigg M, McDermott FT, Pihl EA, Hughes ES. Curative local excision in the treatment of carcinoma of the rectum. *Dis Colon Rectum* 1984;27(2):81–3.
76. Cuthbertson AM, Simpson RL. Curative local excision of rectal adenocarcinoma. *Aust N Z J Surg* 1986;56(3):229–31.
77. Gall FP, Hermanek P. Cancer of the rectum – local excision. *Surg Clin North Am* 1988;68(6):1353–65.
78. Gerard A, Pector JC, Ferreira J. Local excision as conservative treatment for small rectal cancer. *Eur J Surg Oncol* 1989;15(6):544–6.
79. Horn A, Halvorsen JF, Morild I. Transanal extirpation for early rectal cancer. *Dis Colon Rectum* 1989;32:769–772.
80. Benoist S, Panis Y, Martella L, Nemeth J, Hautefeuille P, Valleur P. Local excision of rectal cancer for cure: should we always regard rigid pathologic criteria? *Hepatogastroenterology* 1998;45(23):1546–51.
81. Coco C, Magistrelli P, Granone P, Roncolini G, Picciocchi A. Conservative surgery for early cancer of the distal rectum. *Dis Colon Rectum* 1992;35(2):131–6.
82. Chakravarti A, Compton CC, Shellito PC, Wood WC, Landry J, Machuta SR, et al. Long-term follow-up of patients with rectal cancer managed by local excision with and without adjuvant irradiation. *Ann Surg* 1999;230(1):49–54.
83. Varma MG, Rogers SJ, Schrock TR, Welton ML. Local excision of rectal carcinoma. *Arch Surg* 1999;134(8):863–7; discussion 867–8.
84. Blair S, Ellenhorn JD. Transanal excision for low rectal cancers is curative in early-stage disease with favorable histology. *Am Surg* 2000;66(9):817–20.
85. Balani A, Turoldo A, Braini A, Scaramucci M, Roseano M, Leggeri A. Local excision for rectal cancer. *J Surg Oncol* 2000;74(2):158–62.
86. Mellgren A, Sirivongs P, Rothenberger DA, Madoff RD, Garcia-Aguilar J. Is local excision adequate therapy for early rectal cancer? *Dis Colon Rectum* 2000;43(8):1064–71; discussion 1071–4.
87. Lamont JP, McCarty TM, Digan RD, Jacobson R, Tulanon P, Lichliter WE. Should locally excised T1 rectal cancer receive adjuvant chemoradiation? *Am J Surg* 2000;180(6):402–5; discussion 405–6.
88. Gao JD, Shao YF, Bi JJ, Shi SS, Liang J, Hu YH. Local excision carcinoma in early stage. *World J Gastroenterol* 2003;9(4):871–3.
89. Gopaul D, Belliveau P, Vuong T, Trudel J, Vasilevsky CA, Corns R, et al. Outcome of local excision of rectal carcinoma. *Dis Colon Rectum* 2004;47(11):1780–8.
90. Nascimbeni R, Nivatvongs S, Larson DR, Burgart LJ. Long-term survival after local excision for T1 carcinoma of the rectum. *Dis Colon Rectum* 2004;47(11):1773–9.
91. Bentrem DJ, Okabe S, Wong WD, Guillem JG, Weiser MR, Temple LK, et al. T1 adenocarcinoma of the rectum: transanal excision or radical surgery? *Ann Surg* 2005;242(4):472–7; discussion 477–9.
92. Heintz A, Morschel M, Junginger T. Comparison of results after transanal endoscopic microsurgery and radical resection for T1 carcinoma of the rectum. *Surg Endosc* 1998;12(9):1145–8.
93. Langer C, Liersch T, Markus P, Suss M, Ghadimi M, Fuzesi L, et al. Transanal endoscopic micro-surgery (TEM) for minimally invasive resection of rectal adenomas and "Low-risk" carcinomas (uT1, G1 - 2). *Z Gastroenterol* 2002;40(2):67–72.
94. Lee W, Lee D, Choi S, Chun H. Transanal endoscopic microsurgery and radical surgery for T1 and T2 rectal cancer. *Surg Endosc* 2003;17(8):1283–7.
95. Stipa F, Burza A, Lucandri G, Ferri M, Pigazzi A, Ziparo V, et al. Outcomes for early rectal cancer managed with transanal endoscopic microsurgery: a 5-year follow-up study. *Surg Endosc* 2006;20(4):541–5.
96. Maslekar S, Pillinger SH, Monson JR. Transanal endoscopic microsurgery for carcinoma of the rectum. *Surg Endosc* 2007;21(1):97–102.

Chapter 11
Full-Thickness Local Excision

Lauren A. Kosinski, John H. Marks, and Gerald J. Marks

In 1984 when we first ventured to perform a full-thickness disc excision of a distal rectal cancer after full-dose radiation therapy in an elderly, medically compromised woman, we were filled with wonder. Would the reconstructed radiated rectum heal? Would there be long-term local control of the cancer? In contrast to a radical resection of the rectum following irradiation, where nonirradiated, proximal descending colon is anastomosed to an irradiated rectal remnant, a local excision involves approximation of irradiated tissue.

The foundation for this approach was laid beginning in 1976 when we began administering high-dose neoadjuvant therapy before performing radical proctectomies. The experience we gained operating in the irradiated pelvis emboldened us to adapt this approach for the medically inoperable patient with rectal cancer. The next evolution occurred with the introduction of transanal endoscopic microsurgery (TEM) and our utilization of this technique in patients treated neoadjuvantly.

Introduction

In this chapter, we focus on TEM full-thickness local excision (FTLE) as definitive surgical therapy in rectal cancer patients who have undergone neoadjuvant chemoradiation therapy. In addition to presenting our patient selection scheme and describing the operative technique, we relate the history of our approach and its rationale.

Cancer control is the foremost objective of rectal cancer management, but there are several secondary goals of the *ideal* treatment, including:

- Minimizing morbidity and mortality
- Minimizing patient trauma
- Preserving good bowel function
- Avoiding permanent colostomy

We employ a multimodal rectal cancer treatment approach pioneered by Gerald Marks and Mohamed Mohiuddin, who first delivered preoperative radiation therapy for rectal cancer at Thomas Jefferson University in 1976. This formed the base of the world's first program of sphincter preservation surgery after high-dose radiation therapy [1–5]. This approach is at the intersection of many critical and evolving issues in rectal cancer

---

L.A. Kosinski (✉)
Lankenau, Bryn Mawr, and Paoli Hospitals, Wynnewood, PA, USA

P.A. Cataldo, G.F. Buess (eds.), *Transanal Endoscopic Microsurgery*,
DOI 10.1007/978-0-387-76397-2_11, © Springer Science+Business Media, LLC 2009

management such as the appropriate use of local excision versus radical resection and the role and timing of radiotherapy for tumors of different T-stages and at different levels of the rectum.

Although some centers are examining the role of chemoradiation therapy alone for select, responsive rectal cancers [6–8], meticulous surgical technique remains the cornerstone of rectal cancer care and the major determinant of locoregional control. Local recurrence rates after radical proctectomy decrease when total mesorectal excision is performed [9], and oncologic outcomes improve when practicing surgeons are educated in this technique [10–12]. Radical proctectomy, which is the standard against which other procedures are measured, is still achieved worldwide by abdominoperineal resection 40–60% of the time regardless of rectal cancer level [13–16]. Treatment with radical resection and permanent stoma prevail despite questions about the necessity for this approach in all cases and recognition that the life expectancy of some patients is jeopardized by major abdominal surgery and extensive pelvic dissection.

At the other end of the operative spectrum, FTLE without pelvic irradiation has unacceptably high local failure rates [17–22]. Local excision of T2 cancers without neoadjuvant or adjuvant therapy results in local recurrence rates ranging from 17 to 47%. Even T1 cancers have an appreciable risk of local recurrence ranging from 8 to 29% without chemoradiation therapy [22].

In addition to utilizing neoadjuvant therapy to optimize oncologic outcomes following FTLE, we suspect that the technique of FTLE contributes to local control. Not only does TEM provide access for local excision of lesions in the mid and upper rectum, early evidence suggests TEM enhances oncologic outcomes compared with transanal local excision. The stereoscopic, magnified view of the TEM operating scope combined with rectal insufflation provides superior visualization of rectal tumors. Improved reach and enhanced visualization foster performance of en bloc FTLEs and avoidance of piecemeal resections. Such piecemeal resections violate the tumor, possibly shedding cancer cells into the rectal wound and thereby potentiating higher local recurrence rates.

History

As is often the case in surgical advancement, innovation occurs at the confluence of emerging technology and clinical challenges presented by particular patients. Medically inoperable patients with T3 rectal cancers presented such a dilemma for Marks and Mohiuddin 30 years ago. It was appreciated that good palliation could be achieved with radiation therapy but without durable results. They also recognized that local treatment would fail with all but the most superficial cancers. Even though assessment of lymph node involvement by endorectal ultrasound has improved substantially since the 1970s [23, 24], failure to accurately identify regional nodal metastases is a putative cause of local treatment failure of rectal cancers. Involvement of the perirectal tubular lymphatics as a source of local excision treatment failure was also postulated (and would still be underdiagnosed by endorectal ultrasound). In the late 1970s, Mohiuddin and Marks undertook a program of high-dose neoadjuvant radiation therapy followed by FTLE in 15 medically compromised patients with T3 rectal cancers. In 1994 they reported a 5-year survival of 74% in this group. Two complications were reported (rectal prolapse and rectovaginal fistula). The local recurrence rates based on downstaged tumors were 13% for T0/T1, 0% for T2, and 67% for T3 cancers [1, 25].

These preliminary excellent results led to the extension of the program to 18 medically fit patients with favorable (T1 or T2) rectal cancers who, at the time, would have been candidates for FTLE alone without neoadjuvant therapy. With a mean follow-up of 40 months, the postradiation T2 tumors had a local recurrence rate of 0%, markedly better than previously reported local recurrence rates of 17–47% following FTLE alone for T2 rectal cancers [17–21]. Subsequently, similar improvements of local recurrence rates and 5-year survival were noted in medically *unfit* patients whose T3 tumors regressed to T0 to T2 after neoadjuvant radiation therapy.

Not only were these oncologic outcomes encouraging, there were significant technical implications of these results. This early experience demonstrated that local excision in the irradiated rectum healed successfully and could be performed with minimal morbidity. Furthermore, sphincter function assessed by Parks criteria was excellent in 88% of these patients.

In 1996, John Marks initiated the treatment of rectal cancers by TEM FTLE following neoadjuvant, high-dose chemoradiation therapy. In a 9-year period (1994–2003), 83 patients underwent FTLE after high-dose neoadjuvant radiotherapy. Local recurrence was statistically independent of the type of procedure, but there was a trend suggesting TEM superiority.

In our experience, multimodal therapy enhances the success of local excision in medically compromised patients. We have reported substantial improvement of the local recurrence rate following FTLE of T2 rectal cancers treated neoadjuvantly at a mean follow-up of 63 months: 6% versus 17–47% reported in the literature for T2 cancers treated by FTLE alone. Our treatment algorithm extends the possibility of sphincter preservation by FTLE to select medically fit patients with T1 and T2 cancers.

Patient Selection

Patient selection is key to the success of this approach. Our rectal cancer treatment selection scheme is depicted in Fig. 11.1. We recommend high-dose neoadjuvant chemoradiation therapy for unfavorable cancers (e.g., beyond T2 or node-positive) at all levels of the rectum and for favorable cancers in the distal two thirds of the rectum (0.5–6 cm above

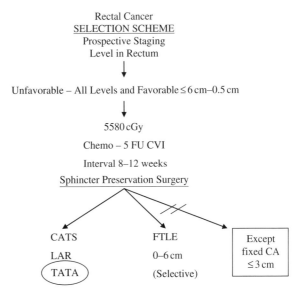

Fig. 11.1 Rectal cancer selection scheme. *5 FU* 5-fluorouracil, *CVI* continuous venous infusion, *CATS* combined abdominotranssacral proctosigmoidectomy, *LAR* low anterior resection, *TATA* transanal abdominal transanal proctosidmoidectomy, *FTLE* full-thickness local excision, *CA* cancer

the anorectal ring). There is a greater risk of local recurrence after resection of low rectal tumors than for those in the more cephalad rectum, and the salvage of recurrences is more difficult owing to early sidewall involvement at this narrowest part of the pelvis. Preoperative chemoradiation therapy is also advised for favorable tumors in the upper third of the rectum in patients deemed high risk for radical resection. Patient selection for FTLE is based on clinical node stage *before* chemoradiation therapy and clinical T-stage *after* neoadjuvant treatment. Endorectal ultrasound and/or pelvic MRI are used to determine node status. FTLE candidates are categorized as either medically compromised or electively staged. Patients electively staged for FTLE are T-stage 2 or less and node-negative. Patients who prove to have pathologic T-stage 3 or greater undergo radical resection unless comorbidities are prohibitive.

Between 1984 and 2003, 83 of 732 rectal cancer patients treated in our practice and entered into a prospectively maintained database underwent FTLE after preoperative radiation therapy. Twenty-nine percent ($n=24$) were medically compromised. Concurrent 5-fluorouracil-based chemotherapy was given to 23 (28%) of the FTLE patients. Two thirds (63%) of the cancers were in the distal 2–cm of the true rectum, and the pretreatment T-stage was 2 or greater in 81% of the patients. With a mean follow-up of 63 months (range 2–226 months), the overall local recurrence rate was 12%. Ten patients had a local recurrence. One of these was salvaged with abdominoperineal resection and is presently without evidence of disease. One patient died of disease. One recurrence (30 months after FTLE) was in a patient with pT2N1 disease who declined radical surgery. The overall 5-year disease-specific survival was 83.3%; it ranged from 80 to 92% for pT0–T2 cancers, and for pT3 cancers it was 53%. The overall Kaplan–Meier 5-year actuarial survival was 78.7%. By conventional standards of practice, 67% of the patients in this group would have had an abdominoperineal resection. Permanent colostomy was avoided in 88% of these patients.

Although there are limited data about TEM in the neoadjuvantly treated rectum, Lezoche et al. [26] reported long-term follow-up (median 52 months) in a group of 20 patients with pretreatment T2N0 rectal tumors. Following high-dose preoperative chemoradiation therapy and TEM excision, the local recurrence rate was just 5%. These data and our own demonstrate that low local recurrence rates can be achieved after FTLE of intermediate T-stage rectal cancer with neoadjuvant therapy. These local recurrence rates are not only lower than expected compared with those of FTLEs performed without neoadjuvant therapy [17–21], they also are the same as or better than the local recurrence rate of 15.1% after standard resection published in a recent retrospective review of 866 T2 cancers [21]. While there has been reluctance to offer radiation therapy to early or intermediate rectal cancer patients, new level I data from the CR07 trial in Great Britain and Ireland indicate that neoadjuvant chemoradiation therapy reduces the local recurrence risk for all T-stages at all levels of the rectum and is superior to adjuvant chemoradiation therapy [27].

Technical Issues

Patients receive 4,500–7,000 cGy with concurrent 5-fluorouracil-based chemotherapy over a 6-week period. We see our patients at 3-week intervals during (and after) neoadjuvant treatment to monitor progress. Most importantly, a visit just before completing radiotherapy helps to determine the need for additional radiation therapy. Tumors that remained fixed or have not responded optimally to treatment may benefit from additional radiation therapy and make *FTLE* by *TEM* possible. *FTLE is reserved for cancers which are post chemoradiated*

11 Full-Thickness Local Excision

T2 or less. If FTLE uncovers a T3 stage, radical resection is advised. The postradiation assessment typically is made 6 weeks after neoadjuvant treatment has been completed. Surgery is performed 8–12 weeks after completion of chemoradiation therapy in order to maximize the tumoricidal effects of treatment.

The technique of TEM has been well described in earlier chapters. Caveats for performing TEM in the irradiated pelvis include the following:

- Fecal diversion is not routinely performed.
- Should fecal diversion be required, transverse loop colostomy is preferred over a loop ileostomy. The terminal ileum is more likely to have been exposed to the radiation field than the transverse colon and would be at greater risk of anastomotic leak at the time of stoma closure or anastomotic stricture at a later date.
- A 14-day course of doxycycline with its collagenase-inhibiting properties and its gram-negative and anaerobic spectrum of coverage may decrease the incidence of postoperative infection in the irradiated rectum.

We have had no perioperative mortalities after FTLE. The morbidity rate was 24% (in 20 patients). The vast majority of these were wound separations (90%). Eighty percent of these were minor and were treated with oral antibiotics; one patient had a temporary colostomy. Two patients had major wound separations that required colostomy diversion, one of which was permanent.

Postoperative Issues

Function in the FTLE group was very good. Although diarrhea and tenesmus were common in the first 24 months postoperatively, these symptoms typically diminish over time. Ninety-three percent of patients were fully continent according to Parks criteria. Fiber supplementation can often resolve functional problems after radiation therapy and FTLE. Selective addition of Lomotil is helpful to some patients. Occasionally, patients who are bothered by clustering of bowel movements will also benefit from hycosamine (Levsyn) taken sublingually.

Follow-Up

Flexible sigmoidoscopy is performed at each 3-month follow-up visit during the first 3 years and at 6-month follow-up for the next 2 years to inspect the anastomosis, which is also palpated when it is within reach of the examining finger. If, as sometimes happens, the silver clips are incorporated into the suture line rather than being shed, they can resemble local recurrence. Any suspicious granulation tissue or nodularity must be evaluated. Sometimes an examination under anesthesia is necessary to fully evaluate and biopsy such sites. Three-tesla MRI and PET scans can augment the evaluation of suspected recurrence. In all patients, full colonoscopy is performed 1 year postoperatively. Carcinoembryonic antigen levels are monitored on the same schedule as office follow-ups; complete blood count, liver function tests, abdominopelvic CT scan, and chest evaluation with X-ray or CT scan are performed annually or as dictated by symptoms or findings on examination. Close follow-up over the long term is essential, especially since the time interval to local recurrence appears to be longer after neoadjuvant treatment, with recurrences noted more than 5 years after.

Conclusion

With a mature experience of 20 years' treatment of rectal cancer with preoperative radiotherapy and FTLE, we have established that FTLE can be accomplished safely after high-dose neoadjuvant chemoradiation therapy. The multimodal approach with FTLE compared with radical proctectomy appears to provide acceptable local control, equivalent survival (including salvage of local failures), satisfactory sphincter function, and durable results. Longer-term follow-up and prospective, randomized trials comparing TEM and transanal approaches with radical proctectomy are needed.

Our success with high-dose chemoradiation therapy before radical resection and local excision of rectal cancers is now being affirmed by large, prospectively randomized trials. In fact, for patients undergoing radical proctectomy, neoadjuvant high-dose chemoradiation therapy has proven oncologically beneficial compared with selectively administered adjuvant therapy for rectal cancers of all T-stages at all levels of the rectum. This benefit has not come at the expense of increased perioperative morbidity or mortality or worse rectal function.

References

1. Mohiuddin M, et al. High-dose preoperative radiation and full thickness local excision: a new option for selected T3 distal rectal cancers. Int J Rad Onc Biol Phys 1994, 30(4): 845–9.
2. Mohiuddin M, et al. A selective sandwich technique of adjuvant radiotherapy in the treatment of rectal cancer: a preliminary experience. Dis Colon Rectum 1979 Jan–Feb, 22(1): 1–4.
3. Marks GJ, et al. Radical sphincter preservation surgery with coloanal anastomosis following high-dose external irradiation for the very low lying rectal cancer. Recent Results Cancer Res 1998, 146: 161–74.
4. Mohiuddin M, et al. High dose preoperative radiation and sphincter preservation in the treatment of rectal cancer. Int J Rad Onc Biol Phys 1987, 13(6): 839–842.
5. Marks GJ, et al. Preoperative radiation therapy and sphincter preservation by the combined abdominotranssacral technique for selected rectal cancers. Dis Colon Rectum 1985, 28(8): 565–571.
6. Habr-Gama A, et al. Operative versus nonoperative treatment for Stage 0 distal rectal cancer following chemoradiation therapy: long-term results. Ann Surg 2004 Oct, 240(4): 711–7.
7. Habr-Gama A, et al. Assessment and management of the complete clinical response of rectal cancer to chemoradiotherapy. Colorectal Dis 2006 Sep; 8 Supp 3: 21–4.
8. Habr-Gama A, et al. Low rectal cancer: impact of radiation and chemotherapy on surgical treatment. Dis Colon Rectum 1998 Sep; 41(9): 1087–96.
9. Heald RJ, et al. Rectal cancer: the Basingstoke experience of total mesorectal excision, 1978–1997. Arch Surg 1998;133(8):894–9.
10. Heald RJ, et al. The 'Holy Plane' of rectal surgery. JR Soc Med 1988 Sep; 81(9): 503–8.
11. Heald RJ, et al. Recurrence and survival after total mesorectal excision or rectal caner. Lancet 1986 Jun 28; 1(8496): 1479–82.
12. Wibe A, et al. Nationwide quality assurance of rectal cancer therapy. Colorect Dis 2006 Mar; 8(3): 224–9.
13. Swedish Rectal Cancer Trial. Improved survival with preoperative radiotherapy in respectable rectal cancer.. N Engl J Med 1997 Apr 3; 336(14): 980–7.
14. Wibe A, et al. Oncologic outcomes after total mesorectal excision for cure of cancer of the lower rectum: anterior vs. abdominoperineal resection. Dis Colon Rectum 2004 Jan; 47(1): 48–58.
15. Kapitijn E, et al. Preoperative radiotherapy combined with total mesorectal excision for resectable rectal cancer N Engl J Med 2001; 345(9): 638–46.
16. Hyams DM, et al. A clinical trial to evaluate the worth of preoperative multimodality therapy in patients with operable carcinoma of the rectum: a progress report of National Surgical Breast and Bowel Project Protocol R-03. Dis Colon Rectum 1997; 40(2): 131–9.
17. Mellgren A, et al. Is local excision adequate therapy for early rectal cancer? Dis Colon Rectum 2000; 43(8): 1064–71.

18. Garcia-Aguilar et al. Local excision of rectal cancer without adjuvant therapy: a word of caution. Ann Surg 2000 Mar; 231(3): 345–51.
19. Taylor RH et al.Transanal local excision of selected low rectal cancers 1998 May; 175(5): 360–3.
20. Paty PB, et al. Long-term results of local excision for rectal cancer. Ann Surg 2002 Oct; 236(4): 522–30.
21. You YN, et al. Is the increasing rate of local excision for stage I rectal cancer in the United States justified?: a nationwide cohort study from the National Cancer Database. Ann Surg 2007 May; 245(5): 726–33.
22. Madbouly KM, et al. Recurrence after transanal excision of T1 rectal cancer: should we be concerned? Dis Colon Rectum 2005 Apr; 248(4): 711–19.
23. Garcia-Aguilar J, et al. Accuracy of endorectal ultrasonography in preoperative staging of rectal tumors. Dis Colon Rectum 2002 Jan; 45(1): 10–5.
24. Schaffzin DM and Wong WD. Endorectal ultrasound in the preoperative evaluation of rectal cancer. Clin Colorectal Cancer. 2004 July; 4(2):124–32.
25. Marks G, et al. High-does preoperative radiation and full thickness local excision: a new option for patients with select cancers of the rectum. Dis Colon Rectum 1990 Sep; 33(9): 735–38.
26. Lezoche E, et al. Transanal endoscopic vs mesorectal laparoscopic resections of T2-N0 low rectal cancers after neoadjuvant therapy. Surg Endose 2005 May; 19:751–756.
27. Srinivasaiah N, et al. How do we manage early rectal cancer? A national questionnaire survey among members of the ACPGBI after the preliminary results of the MRC CR07/NCIC CO16 randomized trial. Colorectal Dis 2008;10(4)357–62.

Chapter 12
Oncologic Outcomes

Joel E. Goldberg and Ronald Bleday

Introduction

Colon and rectal cancer is a major health problem in industrialized societies. In the USA alone there are approximately 145,000 new cases of colorectal cancer per year and approximately 42,000 of these patients are diagnosed with rectal cancer. Moreover, colon and rectal cancer is the third most common cancer diagnosis and the second leading cause of cancer death in both men and women in North America. In fact, 40,000–50,000 deaths can be attributed to colon and rectal cancer each year in the USA alone [1, 2]. A new diagnosis of rectal cancer is very worrisome for many patients because of the need for radical surgery and its potential side effects and consequences. Alterations in bowel and bladder function, sexual dysfunction and, most importantly, the possibility of radical surgery resulting in the need for a permanent colostomy all weigh heavily on the minds of patients diagnosed with rectal cancer.

Locally advanced tumors of the mid and distal rectum (stage II and III disease) are best treated with neoadjuvant chemoradiotherapy followed by either low anterior resection (LAR) or abdominoperineal resection (APR) with permanent colostomy. Since the advent of total mesorectal excision, acceptable rates of local recurrence have been reported for locally advanced cancers [3]. The addition of neoadjuvant chemoradiotherapy to total mesorectal excision has resulted in decreased local recurrence and increased sphincter preservation [4, 5].

Patients with early-stage lesions of the rectum can in some cases be offered less radical surgery through a transanal approach. Improved staging techniques such as endorectal ultrasound and endorectal MRI have allowed for the selection of patients who might be candidates for a less "radical approach" [6].

Many factors play a role in the decision whether to treat a patient suffering from rectal cancer with radical surgery or local excision. The treatment options need to balance the long-term survival and recurrence rates against morbidity and functional results. For stage I cancer there are three surgical options which can then be combined with combinations of adjuvant or neoadjuvant therapy. Two of the three options to consider are radical resection for early disease by either APR or LAR. APR is generally reserved for patients with direct extension of the tumor into the sphincter complex or pre-existing incontinence in which a LAR would only further decrease poor anorectal function. Both LAR and APR result in complete removal of the entire mesorectum. Total mesorectal excision for rectal cancer, popularized by Heald, has resulted in local recurrence rates as low as 4% in curative intent surgery [7]. The rationale for complete excision of the mesorectum is to remove all lymph

---

J.E. Goldberg (✉)
Brigham and Women's Hospital, Harvard Medical School, Boston, MA, USA

P.A. Cataldo, G.F. Buess (eds.), *Transanal Endoscopic Microsurgery*,
DOI 10.1007/978-0-387-76397-2_12, © Springer Science+Business Media, LLC 2009

nodes, extramural tumor deposits contained within the mesorectal fascia and to achieve negative surgical margins. With stage I disease all lymph nodes by definition will be negative for cancer and the tumor will be confined to the rectal wall. The disadvantages of the radical resection are sexual and/or bladder dysfunction in 15–50% of patients, intraoperative bleeding, perioperative medical problems such as myocardial infarction and a mortality rate of approximately 1–2% (historically it has been as high as 6%) [8–11]. However, the main disadvantage of the radical resection is the possible need for a temporary or permanent ostomy and evacuation and/or anorectal dysfunction such as incontinence. Also, recurrence and survival rates with radical surgery are not necessarily improved in the treatment of stage I cancers when compared with those for local excision combined with adjuvant therapy in selected cases. It is with these concepts in mind that we will discuss the oncologic outcomes of transanal endoscopic microsurgery (TEM) for stage I rectal cancer and compare them with those of the traditional transanal excision and radical surgery.

Historical Background

In the late nineteenth and early twentieth centuries local excision of rectal tumors was commonplace as there was no alternative until Miles popularized APR in the early twentieth century. Prior to Miles's description of APR, there was little knowledge of the natural history of rectal cancer; therefore, local excision appeared to be most prudent technique to remove a rectal cancer. However, in 1908 Miles observed high recurrence rates in patients following local excision. As an alternative, he developed his radical APR, which has become known as the Miles resection [12]. It was believed that radical resections such as Miles's APR provided the best opportunity for cure, and this radical resection quickly became the standard of care despite its increased morbidity and mortality compared with local excisions. Over the ensuing decades, despite improvements in the morbidity and mortality, both surgeons and patients alike looked for alternatives to radical rectal cancer surgery that would avoid a permanent colostomy [13]. In 1977, Morson et al. reported the results from St. Mark's Hospital in London of the treatment of early-stage distal rectal cancers using a transanal approach [33]. As a result, local excision of rectal tumors was once again advocated by many surgeons for early-stage rectal cancer with favorable histologic criteria.

In the medically fit patient the standard indications for curative intent transanal local excision of rectal carcinoma include a location with 8 cm of the anal verge, tumor size less than 4 cm (or less than one third the circumference of the rectal lumen), node-negative T1 or T2 lesions by endorectal ultrasound or MRI with endorectal coil, well to moderately differentiated tumors with no lymphovascular or perineural invasion and nonmucinous tumors [14]. Several technical aspects of transanal excision of rectal cancers make this procedure challenging and of limited use. The narrow anal canal and the bony confines of the pelvis make it difficult to resect tumors more proximal than 8 cm from the anal verge. With this in mind, in 1980 Gerhard Buess of Tübingen, Germany, began developing a system for TEM that would enable the operating surgeon to resect rectal tumors and polyps in the middle and upper rectum [15]. Over the last 27 years TEM has become widely used in Europe, but has been slower to develop in North America; however, in recent years momentum has increased and TEM is now becoming standard practice for many surgeons performing local excision. The indications for TEM are the same as for traditional transanal local excision with the one major exception and advantage that TEM allows the surgeon to operate on lesions anywhere within the rectum [16, 17].

Preoperative Assessment

Preoperative evaluation includes a thorough history and physical with specific attention being paid to note sphincter function as local excision in the setting of poor sphincter function is inappropriate. A digital rectal examination helps determine the distance of the tumor from the anal verge in addition to its size and mobility. In order to perform either a traditional transanal local excision or a TEM procedure the patient must be accurately staged. The abovementioned history and physical are the first steps in determining who is a good candidate for local excision. Either technique may be utilized in patients who are unfit for major abdominal surgery or in patients with widely metastatic disease who require surgical palliation of a symptomatic primary tumor. However, in the medically fit patient who is undergoing curative intent surgery accurate assessment of the preoperative stage is of paramount importance as the T stage, N stage (lymph node status) and histologic features all play a significant role in the decision whether to pursue local excision. After the history and physical, further investigation is warranted with a complete colonoscopy with biopsy of the lesion in question and any synchronous lesions. Second, T stage and lymph node staging with either endorectal ultrasound or endorectal coil MRI must be performed. Once an accurate assessment has been made and the patient has been staged as having lymph node negative T1 or T2 disease either anal technique can be utilized for curative intent resection. Accurate T and N staging is critical to successful local excision by either technique.

Removing all involved lymph nodes is equally as important as achieving a negative radial margin. Many studies have shown a strong correlation between lymph node metastases and the primary tumor's depth of invasion into the bowel wall. Nascimbeni et al. [18] reported that T1 carcinoma is associated with positive lymph nodes in 13% of cases. Sitzler et al. [19] reported that 5.7% of T1 lesions, 19.6% of T2 lesions, 65.7% of T3 lesions and 78.8% of T4 lesions have lymph node metastases. Moreover, several studies have reported histopathologic predictors of LN metastases in rectal cancers. Poor differentiation, lymphovascular invasion, perineural invasion and lesions in the lower third of the rectum are strongly associated with a higher degree of lymph node metastases [20]. Poor histopathologic features and the increased chance of lymph node metastases with more advanced T stage both play a critical role in the decision of whether to treat a patient with a low-lying rectal cancer with local excision. Despite being a frequently utilized technique for early-stage rectal cancers, traditional local excision has been highly criticized for high rates of local recurrence. Conversely, early reports with TEM have been favorable with respect to oncologic outcomes and relatively low rates of local recurrence.

Technique

There are four approaches to local excision of rectal cancer: transanal, transcoccygeal, transsphincteric and TEM. We will focus our discussion and description on the traditional transanal excision and TEM.

Transanal Excision

Local excision can be accomplished via a transanal approach for the majority of low rectal cancers. In preparation for surgery all patients should receive a full mechanical bowel preparation. Depending on the location of the lesion, the patient is placed in either the prone-jackknife position or the lithotomy position with the buttocks taped apart. A pudendal nerve block should be given as it will aid in postoperative pain control and intraoperatively will help to relax the sphincter complex. The anal canal is then dilated and a handheld retractor such as a Pratt bivalve and/or a self-retaining retractor such as a Lone Star retractor is used to help with the exposure. Most surgeons utilize traction sutures to help with the exposure as well. The sutures should be placed 2 cm distal to the tumor and then a circumferential line of dissection is mapped out on the mucosa using electrocautery. This line of dissection should be approximately 1 cm from the border of the tumor circumferentially. Electrocautery is then used to perform a full-thickness excision of the lesion into the underlying perirectal fat along the demarcated mucosa. If possible, the defect in the bowel wall should be closed transversely with interrupted absorbable 3-0 sutures.

Transanal Endoscopic Microsurgery

The surgery is performed using a special 4-cm-diameter operating proctoscope which is available in lengths of 12 and 20 cm. After the patient has been appropriately positioned so that the lesion is towards the floor, the anal canal is gently dilated. The operating procto-scope is then inserted and an airtight glass faceplate replaces the obturator. The scope is then secured to the operating table with the aid of a support arm. The glass faceplate is replaced with a working faceplate that contains three instrument ports and a camera port. Carbon dioxide is then insufflated anywhere from 10–15 cm H_2O pressure in order to distend the rectum and allow for the operation to be performed. The operative technique proceeds very similarly to a transanal excision. Special endoscopic instruments are introduced through the working ports and are used to excise the tumor. Once again, the margin of resection is marked 1 cm circumferentially around the lesion using electrocautery. After the marking is completed, the mucosa just distal to the lesion is grasped and the excision proceeds along the previously marked line. Just as in a transanal excision, the dissection is carried down through the full thickness of the rectal wall and into the perirectal fat. The specimen is removed and pinned out for the pathologist to evaluate the margins and the defect is then closed transversely using interrupted 3-0 polydioxanone sutures in a figure-of-eight or running fashion.

Outcomes

Transanal Local Excision

The vast majority of the literature for local excision of rectal cancer by either transanal excision or TEM comes from single institution small retrospective reviews. As can be expected, these studies are difficult to interpret because there is no uniform approach to gathering, analyzing and interpreting the data. Many of these studies compare local excision with radical surgery with or without adjuvant therapy. Moreover, the follow-up varies between the studies as do the follow up parameters.

12 Oncologic Outcomes

Table 12.1 Local excision with and without radiotherapy

Series authors	No. of patients	Follow-up (years)	Local recurrence	Survival
Nascimbeni et al. [25]	70 (T1)	8.1 (median)	T1 7%	T1 89% (cancer-specific survival)
Paty et al. [24]	74 (T1) 51 (T2)	6.7 (median)	T1 17%[a] T2 26%[a]	T1 74% (disease-specific)[a] T2 72% (disease-specific)[a]
Garcia-Aguilar et al. [22]	55 (T1) 27 (T2)	4.5 (average)	T1 16% (local + distant = 18%) T2 30% (local + distant = 37%)	T1 77% (overall survival after salvage surgery) T2 55% (overall survival after salvage surgery)
Mellgren et al. [21]	69 (T1) 39 (T2)	4.4 (mean)	T1 18% (estimated) T2 47% (estimated)	T1 72% (overall survival rate) T2 65% (overall survival rate)
Bleday et al. [23]	21 (T1) 21 (T2) 5 (T3)	3.4 (mean)	T1 9.5% T2 0%[a] T3 40%[a]	Overall 93.8%

[a] Includes patients who received adjuvant radiotherapy

For traditional transanal excision, the largest and most recent retrospective reviews report local recurrence rates of 7–18% for T1 tumors and 26–47% for T2 tumors without adjuvant therapy. Overall and cancer-specific survival rates range from 72 to 89% for T1 lesions and from 55 to 72% for T2 lesions (Table 12.1) [21–25]. In the studies by Garcia-Aguilar et al. [22], Nascimbeni et al. [25] and Mellgren et al. [21] all of the patients had negative margins, favorable histologic features, full-thickness excision and no adjuvant therapy. In the study of Bleday et al. [23] all T2 and T3 patients received adjuvant radiotherapy and in the study of Paty et al. some patients received adjuvant therapy. In study of Paty et al. [24], the overall local recurrence did not change between those patients treated with radiation and those treated without radiation; however, the time to recurrence was longer in those who received adjuvant therapy. These studies demonstrate that superficial tumors (T1 lesions) with negative margins and favorable histologic features can have low rates of local recurrence and survival similar to patients who have had radical resection. These studies suggest that local excision may provide adequate oncologic control for early lesions with much lower morbidity and mortality than an APR. In fact, a recent meta-analysis looking at studies utilizing local excision and APR for distal rectal cancers as well as data from the National Cancer Database (NCDB) showed no difference in overall survival in a comparison of APR versus local excision for T1N0 and T2N0 lesions. In this study, patients with T1 lesions treated by local excision had 83% overall survival versus 73% overall survival for those who had an APR. Patients with T2 lesions also showed no difference, with local excision patients having 80% overall survival and those getting an APR having 69% overall survival. The NCDB data confirmed these findings as patients with T1 and T2 lesions treated with local excision had 76 and 74.9% overall survival and all patients with stage I (T1N0 and T2N0) lesions treated with APR had an overall survival of 73%. None of these differences were statistically significant [26].

Transanal Endoscopic Microsurgery

The literature about TEM resection of rectal cancers is from small series at single institutions with short-term follow-up. These studies often directly compare TEM resection with radical resection with favorable morbidity and mortality but never directly make a comparison with traditional transanal resection. Local recurrence for low-risk T1 adenocarcinoma of the rectum resected by TEM ranges from 0 to 11% and local recurrence for T2 lesions without adjuvant therapy ranges from 19.5 to 35%. The addition of adjuvant or neoadjuvant therapy to treatment of T2 and T3 lesions combined with TEM shows local recurrence rates of 14 and 3%, respectively (Table 12.2) [27–32]. The follow-up in these studies, however, is relatively short, with the longest reported follow-up being 4 years.

An indirect comparison of the local recurrence rates for transanal resection with those for TEM shows that for T1 lesions with favorable histologic features the expected local recurrence rates should be 7–18% and 0–11%, respectively. These are comparable results and it can be assumed that in a medically fit patient with a T1 rectal adenocarcinoma that either a TEM resection or a traditional transanal excision is acceptable and that the decision as to which should be utilized rests more with the location of the tumor and the skill set of the individual surgeon. On the other hand, local recurrence rates for transanal excision and for TEM for T2 lesions are 26–47% and 19.5–35%, respectively. Neither of these is satisfactory. The addition of radiotherapy to the treatment of T2 lesions significantly lowers the local recurrence rate for both TEM and transanal excision. However, in the medically fit patient in which the intent is curative neither TEM nor transanal excision can be recommended alone as the sole mode of treatment.

To satisfactorily answer this question, it will be necessary to have a multi-institutional study comparing side by side the surgical treatment of stage I rectal cancer by TEM versus transanal excision alone for T1 lesions and the same for T2 lesions with the addition of either adjuvant or neoadjuvant chemoradiotherapy. It is our opinion that TEM will have a better outcome than traditional transanal excision for three main reasons. First, TEM is utilized for lesions located more proximally in the rectum. It is generally accepted that

Table 12.2 Transanal endoscopic microsurgery (*TEM*) with and without radiotherapy

Series Authors	No. of patients	Follow-up	Local recurrence	Survival
Borschitz et al. [30]	37 (T2; 20 patients TEM alone, 17 radical surgery after TEM) operated on for cure	TEM alone 3.8 years (median) TEM + radical surgery 8.9 years (median)	TEM alone T2 35% (29% in low-risk TEM) TEM + radical surgery 12% local and 12% distant recurrence	
Maslekar et al. [29]	27 (T1) 25 (T2, T3)	3.3 years (mean)	T1 0% (no adjuvant therapy) T2, T3 14% (adjuvant therapy)	
Floyd and Saclarides [32]	37 (T1)	3.3 years (mean)	T1 11%	
Lee et al. [27]	52 (T1) 22 (T2)		T1 4.1% T2 19.5%	
Lezoche et al. [28]	35 (T2; all had neoadjuvant therapy)	3.2 years (median)	T2 3%	Survival at 96 months, 83%
Buess [31]	108 (T1)	4.3 years (mean)	T1 5%	

rectal cancers located in the distal third of the rectum (those accessible by traditional transanal resection) have a poorer prognosis than those located in the proximal two thirds of the rectum (lesions accessible by TEM). Second, TEM offers better visualization of the lesion and, as a result, a more complete resection of the margins within the lumen of the rectum. Finally, and most importantly, TEM allows for better visualization of the radial resection margin within the perirectal fat.

Conclusions

The treatment of early-stage rectal cancer has come full circle over the last two centuries. Initially, local excision was utilized because of a poor understanding of the natural history of rectal cancer and the inability of medical professionals to provide the supportive care necessary for patients undergoing major oncologic resections. After Miles popularized the APR, radical surgery became the standard for almost 50 years. Currently local excision has slowly made a comeback as a reaction to the morbidity and mortality of the radical resections. Both traditional transanal excision and TEM have acceptable results for favorable T1 lesions, with a trend toward TEM having lower local recurrence rates. For T2 lesions, both techniques carry an unacceptably high local recurrence rate without the addition of adjuvant chemoradiation therapy. In the end, we must remember that to date there is no direct comparison of these two techniques, and as a result the skill set of the surgeon and the accessibility of the tumor often determine the surgical technique.

Editor's Note

At the University of Vermont we have compared TEM with standard transanal excision for the treatment of rectal cancers and polyps in 171 patients (J. Moore and P.A. Cataldo, unpublished data; presented at ASCRS St. Louis, June 2007). TEM is significantly more likely to result in excisions of intact, nonfragmented specimens (94 vs 65%, $p<0.001$). In addition, tumor-free margins were significantly more likely following TEM (98 vs 78%, $p=0.01$, in malignancy and 83 vs 61% in benign polyps, $p=0.03$).

Recurrence rates following curative resection were also better after TEM than after transanal excision (TEM 3%, transanal excision 22% for malignancy; TEM 3%, transanal excision 32% for benign polyps). These numbers, however, did not reach statistical significance owing to small sample size. At 3-year follow-up, overall mortality was 2% in the TEM group compared with 29% in the transanal excision group ($p=0.01$). In addition, the morbidity was similar in both groups.

These results, in a moderate-size study, indicate that TEM is technically superior to transanal excision and appears to be associated with better oncologic outcomes. These results await publication and validation by further studies.

References

1. Cancer Facts and Statistics 2004. Atlanta: American Cancer Society.
2. Jemal A, Murray T, Samuela A, et al. Cancer statistics, 2003. CA Cancer J Clin 2003;53:5.
3. Heald RJ, Moran BJ, Ryall, RD, et al. Rectal cancer: The Basingstoke experience of total mesorectal excision, 1978–1997. Arch Surg 1998;133:894–899.

4. Kapiteijn E, Marijnen CA, Nagtegaal ID, et al. Preoperative radiotherapy combined with total mesorectal excision for resectable rectal cancer. N Engl J Med 2001;345(9):638–646.
5. Sauer R, Becker H, Hohenberger W, et al. Preoperative versus postoperative chemoradiotherapy for rectal cancer. N Engl J Med 2004;351(17):1731–1740.
6. Blumberg D, Paty PB, Picon Ai, et al. Stage I rectal cancer: identification of high-risk patients. J Am Coll Surg 1998;186:574–580.
7. Heald RJ. Rectal cancer: the surgical options. Eur J Cancer 1995;31A(7/8):1189–1192.
8. Rothenberger DA, Wong WD. Abdominoperineal resection for adenocarcinoma of the low rectum. World J Surg 1992; 16(3):478–485.
9. Wong CS, Stern H, Cummings BJ. Local excision and post-operative radiation therapy for rectal carcinoma. Int J Radiat Oncol Biol Phys 1993; 25(4):669–675.
10. Rosen L, Veidenheimer MC, Coller JA, Corman ML. Mortality, morbidity, and patterns of recurrence after abdominoperineal resection for cancer of the rectum. Dis Colon Rectum 1982;25(3):202–208.
11. Pollard CW, Nivatvongs S, Rojanasakul A, Ilstrup DM. Carcinoma of the rectum. Profiles of intraoperative and early postoperative complications. Dis Colon Rectum 1994;37(9):866–874.
12. Miles WE. A method of performing abdomino-perineal excision for carcinoma of the rectum and of the terminal portion of the pelvic colon (1908). CA Cancer J Clin 1971;21(6):361–364.
13. Lock MR. Fifty years of local excision for rectal carcinoma. Ann R Coll Surg Eng 1990;72:170–171.
14. Moore HG, Guillem JG. Local therapy for rectal cancer. Surg Clin N Am 2002;82:967–981.
15. Buess G. Review: transanal endoscopic microsurgery (TEM). J R Coll Surg Edin 1993;38:239–245.
16. Cataldo PA. Transanal endoscopic microsurgery. Surg Clin N Am 2006;86:915–925.
17. Desmartines N, von Flue MO, Harder FH. Transanal endoscopic microsurgical excision of rectal tumors: indications and results. World J Surg 2001;25:870–875.
18. Nascimbeni R, Burgart LJ, Nivatvongs S, Larson DR. Risk of lymph node metastasis in T1 carcinoma of the colon and rectum. Dis Colon Rectum 2002;45:200–206.
19. Sitzler PJ, Seow-Choen F, Ho YH, Leong APK. Lymph node involvement and tumor depth in rectal cancers: an analysis of 805 patients. Dis Colon Rectum 1997;40:1472–1476.
20. Saclarides TJ, Bhattacharyya AK, Britton-Kuzel C, Szeluga D, Economou SG. Predicting lymph node metastases in rectal cancer. Dis Colon Rectum 1994;37:52–57.
21. Mellgren A, Sirivongs P, Rothenberger DA, Madoff RD, Garcia-Aguilar J. Is local excision adequate therapy for early rectal cancer? Dis Colon Rectum 2000;43:1064–1074.
22. Garcia-Aguilar J, Mellgren A, Sirivongs P, Buie D, Madoff RD, Rothenberger DA. Local excision of rectal cancer without adjuvant therapy. A word of caution. Ann Surg 2000;231(3):345–351.
23. Bleday RB, Breen E, Jessup JM, Burgess A, Sentovich Sm, Steele G. Prospective evaluation of local excision for small rectal cancers. Dis Colon Rectum 1997;40:388–392.
24. Paty PB, Nash GM, Baron P, et al. Long-term results of local excision for rectal cancer. Ann Surg 2002;236(4):522–530.
25. Nascimbeni R, Nivatvongs S, Larson DR, Burgart LJ. Long-term survival after local excision for T1 carcinoma of the rectum. Dis Colon Rectum 2004;47:1773–1779.
26. Greenberg J, Lipsitz S, Greenberg C, Bleday R. (unpublished results).
27. Lee W, Lee D, Choi S, Chun H. Transanal endoscopic microsurgery and radical surgery for T1 and T2 rectal cancer. Surg Endosc 2003;17(8):1283–1287.
28. Lezoche E, Guerrieri M, Paganini AM, Feliciotti F. Long-term results of patients with pT2 rectal cancer treated with radiotherapy and transanal endoscopic microsurgical excision. World J Surg 2002;26:1170–1174.
29. Maslekar S, Pillinger SH, Monson JRT. Transanal endoscopic microsurgery for carcinoma of the rectum. Surg Endosc 2006;21:97–102.
30. Borschitz T, Heintz A, Junginger T. Transanal endoscopic microsurgical excision of pT2 rectal cancer: results and possible indications. Dis Colon Rectum 2007;50:292–301.
31. Buess G. Transanal endoscopic microsurgery. Surg Oncol Clin N Am 2001;10:709–731.
32. Floyd ND, Saclarides TJ. Transanal endoscopic microsurgical resection of pT1 rectal tumours. Dis Colon Rectum 2005;49:164–168.
33. Morson BC, Bussey HJ, Samoorian S. Policy of local excision for early cancer of the colorectum. Gut. 1977;18:1045–1050.

Chapter 13
Clinical Trials

Kim F. Rhoads and Julio E. Garcia-Aguilar

Background

Total mesorectal excision (TME) is accepted today as the standard surgical therapy for rectal cancer. Tumors located in the middle or upper third of the rectum can be removed with a restorative anterior resection or low anterior resection (LAR), while those in the lower third have been historically treated with abdominoperineal resection. These aggressive surgical approaches adhere to the successful paradigm of wide resection with a diagnostic and possibly therapeutic lymphadenectomy. Owing to the radical nature of these operations, however, they can and do result in significant mortality, morbidity [1–3] and functional disturbances [4, 5].

Local excision, whether performed by the conventional transanal approach or by transanal endoscopic microsurgery (TEM), is a less invasive alternative approach to the treatment of early rectal cancer. While local excision can be potentially curative for tumors limited to the rectal wall, recent series have reported high rates of local recurrence [6–11]. Patients who fail local excision can in theory be salvaged by radical surgery, but recent data seem to indicate that local excision may compromise survival as compared with radical surgery. Unfortunately there is a very limited body of robust data regarding local excision, as the majority of it derives from case series and retrospective reviews of institutional experiences.

There are a number of logistical and ethical barriers to the design of prospective trials on the use of local excision for the treatment of rectal cancer. Some surgeons will consider it unethical to offer an operation that has been associated with a high rate of recurrence to a patient with a rectal tumor that is curable by an operation that has withstood the test of time. From the patients' perspective, some may not agree to be randomized to one of two different modes of therapy whose results vary so dramatically with regard to changes of body image and functional outcome. From the standpoint of rational study design, the overall survival in patients with stage I rectal cancer treated by either radical surgery or local excision is excellent. Therefore, any study attempting to show significant improvement compared with standardized outcomes would require large numbers of subjects to demonstrate any difference with an acceptable level of statistical power. Finally, surgeons often have strong preferences regarding technical issues and may not agree to randomize patients to two different approaches to the same operation as would occur in any study comparing conventional transanal excision with TEM. With these limitations in mind, we review the prospective studies that have been published so far, and those that are now open for accrual.

K.F. Rhoads (✉)
Mt. Zion Cancer Center, University of California, San Francisco, San Francisco, CA, USA

P.A. Cataldo, G.F. Buess (eds.), *Transanal Endoscopic Microsurgery*,
DOI 10.1007/978-0-387-76397-2_13, © Springer Science+Business Media, LLC 2009

Prospective Trials on Local Excision

The Radiation Therapy Oncology Group (RTOG) conducted a phase II multi-institutional trial of local excision with or without chemoradiation therapy in patients with clinically mobile rectal cancer located below the peritoneal reflection, in which the alternative would be an abdominoperineal excision of the rectum. Patients in this trial had tumors located within 10 cm from the anal verge, less than 4 cm in diameter, involving less than 40% of the circumference of the rectum, and were free of regional metastasis as judged by palpation or pelvic CT scan. Surgical technique called for full-thickness removal with negative margins. Of the 72 patients registered into this protocol, seven were ineligible because of incomplete excision or other reasons, leaving 65 patients for analysis [12]. On the basis of the final histopathological findings, patients were divided into three groups. The first group consisted of 14 patients with a T1 lesion who had favorable histological features and secure margins. This group received no further treatment after surgery and was observed. The second group included 18 patients with T1 tumors and unfavorable histological features or lesions measured at T2 or greater, excised with microscopically negative margins. These patients received postoperative adjuvant therapy with 50–56 Gy of radiation and two cycles of 96 h of continuous intravenous infusion of 5-fluorouracil. The third group included 33 patients with microscopically positive or unsecured margins who were assigned to the same adjuvant therapy but with a boost that increased the dose of radiation to 59.4–65 Gy. A total of 11 patients (16%) developed cancer recurrence or progression at a median of 6.1 years. Ultimately eight patients developed distant metastasis, accompanied or preceded by local recurrence; three patients developed isolated local recurrence. Five patients underwent salvage radical surgery, but four of these patients developed distant recurrence. Actuarial 5-year survival for the entire group was 88%, and 86% for patients who had radiation therapy and chemotherapy. Acute grade 3 or 4 toxicity was reported in 27% of patients who received chemoradiation therapy. The risk of recurrence correlated with increasing T stage and the extent of involvement of the circumference of the rectum, but the study was underpowered and the differences between groups were not significant. In spite of these limitations the authors concluded that local excision alone was a viable option in patients with T1 cancers with favorable histological features, while patients with T2 tumors could be safely treated with local excision followed by chemoradiation therapy. Although not associated with higher rates of recurrences, the poor compliance with surgical guidelines and the high rate of patients with positive resection margins was considered unacceptable.

The Cancer and Leukemia Group B (CALGB) conducted a phase II prospective multi-institutional trial investigating whether survival of patients with stage I rectal cancer treated with local excision was comparable to that of historical controls treated with radical surgery [13]. Patients with biopsy-proven adenocarcinoma of the rectum, located within 10 cm of the anal verge, measuring 4 cm or less in diameter, and involving less than 40% of the circumference on the rectum, were entered into the trial. All patients underwent a battery of tests to exclude nodal disease or distant metastasis. A total of 161 patients underwent full-thickness excision of the tumor by transanal, transphincteric or transcoccygeal approach. A second registration was required after the surgical excision. Tumors with less than full-thickness excision, positive or unclear margins, deeper than a T2 or more superficial than a T1 tumor, and reports without complete information were excluded. In total, 51 patients were excluded, leaving 110 T1 or T2 patients who met all the clinical and histological eligibility criteria. Patients with T1 tumors were observed, while patients with

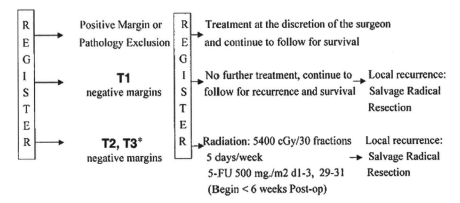

Fig. 13.1 Cancer and Leukemia Group B phase II Clinical Trial for local excision of rectal cancer with or without postoperative chemoradiation. *5-FU* 5-fluorouracil. (From Fig. 1 of Steele et al. [13], with kind permission of Springer Science+Business Media)

T2 tumors received postoperative adjuvant chemoradiation therapy (Fig. 13.1). Two patients with T1 tumors and seven with T2 tumors underwent salvage abdominoperineal excision of the rectum. There was no surgery-related mortality, and morbidity was minimal. Five patients had wound-related complications and four had urinary dysfunction. More than one third of the patients had grade 3 or 4 hematological or gastrointestinal toxicity attributable to the chemoradiation therapy. The estimated 6-year failure-free survival rate for T1 patients was 83%, and for T2 patients it was 71%. The results for all the T1/T2 eligible patients were comparable with those published by the National Cancer Database for stage I patients.

The CALGB study demonstrated that local excision is significantly less morbid than radical surgery and that local excision of T1 and T2 rectal cancer shows no significant therapeutic disadvantage compared with historical data from the National Cancer Database. However, at the time of the last report, a plateau in disease-free survival had not yet been reached, and any additional recurrence could change the conclusions of the study. The exclusion of 51 of the 161 patients who met the entry criteria due mainly to lack of documentation, incomplete excision or transmural invasion raises questions about the possibility of performing an adequate local excision even in the context of a defined protocol. As ineligible patients were not included in the final analysis, the biological implication of such a high rate of exclusion is not clear.

Prospective Trials on TEM

There are two published randomized phase III controlled trials on TEM, as the modality of local excision, for various forms of radical resection for rectal cancers [14–16].

In 1996, Winde et al. [14] prospectively randomized 52 patients with uT1uN0 rectal cancer to either TEM ($n = 26$) or LAR ($n = 24$). Two patients were excluded from the study for unclear reasons. Apparently patients with tumors other than pT1 and/or poorly differentiated histological features were excluded from the study, but the exact number of patients excluded was not explicitly stated. At a mean follow-up of 46 months, there was no significant difference in the local recurrence rate (4.2% for TEM versus 0% for LAR) or survival rate (96% in both arms) with a nonsignificant hazard ratio for death after local excision of 1.02 [15]. TEM was superior in terms of length of surgery, blood loss, hospital stay and analgesic demand. Surgical complications were more frequent after anterior resection (35%) than after TEM (21%), but the differences were not significant. Overall, the authors concluded that TEM for patients with T1 lesions provides comparable oncological outcomes to those of radical surgery. Unfortunately, the sample size was small, leaving the study, though promising, grossly underpowered.

In 2005, Lezoche et al. [15] reported their results of 40 patients with biopsy-proven, grade 1–2, ultrasound-staged T2N0 low-lying adenocarcinoma of the rectum. Distant disease was excluded by a variety of tests. All patients received preoperative radiation therapy (50.4 Gy in 25 fractions over 5 weeks) and continuous infusion of 5-fluorouracil during the course of radiation therapy. After completion of the chemoradiation therapy, patients were randomized to receive TEM or laparoscopic anterior resections involving TME. There were no differences in patient characteristics between groups. At a median follow-up period of 56 months, there were equal numbers of local and distant failures in both arms. The probability of local and distant failure at the end of follow-up was estimated at 10% for the TEM group and 12% for the laparoscopic resection group, corresponding to a nonsignificant relative risk estimate of 1.08 (confidence interval 0.15–7.78). The probability of survival at the end of 78 months was estimated at 95% for the local excision group and 83% for the laparoscopic resection group, a statistically nonsignificant difference. In further support of the benefits of local excision, the authors demonstrated significant clinical advantages in the TEM arm. Patients who underwent TEM had significant decreases in operative time, blood loss, postoperative analgesic requirements and length of stay as compared with the laparoscopic/radical resection group [16].

The authors presented an updated abstract at the 2006 annual meeting of the Society for Surgery of the Alimentary Tract [16]. By this time, they had increased enrollment, having randomized 35 patients into either arm of the study. At a mean follow-up of 68 months for the entire cohort, there were still no significant differences in local recurrence rates (5.7% in the TEM arm versus 2.9% in the laparoscopic arm), or in the incidence of metastatic disease (2.9% in both arms). The authors fortified their conclusions reported in 2005, asserting that TEM appears to be a safe effective treatment of selected T2 carcinomas of the rectum [16].

Neither the study of Winde et al. nor the studies of Lezoche et al. measured functional outcomes after local versus radical resection. There is one study in the current body of literature that compared pre- and postoperative functional outcome after local excision by TEM [17]. The authors found that in spite of the necessary rectal insufflations and instrumentation involved in the TEM procedure, there was no statistically significant change in pre- and postoperative fecal incontinence quality of life scores or symptom index; no change in the number of bowel movements in a 24-h period, or the ability to defer defecation [17]. In this study, patients served as their own controls. To date, there are no prospective randomized trials comparing functional morbidity or specific aspects of oncological outcomes in patients undergoing local versus radical resection.

Current Clinical Trials

In spite of the abundant interest in local excision and TEM, evidenced by a large body of literature, an extensive Web search of US federal and regional cancer Web sites [18–22] reveals limited availability of ongoing clinical trials comparing local and radical excision for rectal cancer. Currently, there is one prospective, nonrandomized, phase II trial to evaluate the local resectability of T2N0 rectal cancers treated with neoadjuvant chemoradiation therapy. The trial is a multicenter effort administered through the American College of Surgeons Oncology Group (ACOSOG) and sponsored by the National Cancer Institute. The study is currently open to patients with uT2uN0 rectal cancers who can tolerate the standardized neoadjuvant therapy regimen. Patients will undergo conventional transanal excision or TEM. The primary outcome in this trial is disease-free survival. This study has a number of secondary aims related to the effect of chemoradiation therapy in early rectal cancer, such as the rate of response to chemoradiation therapy, the impact of chemoradiation therapy on surgical complications after local excision, and the combined effect of chemoradiation therapy and local excision in anorectal function and quality of life. Compliance with surgical guidelines was one of the main criticisms of the RTOG and CALGB trials. The ACOSOG Z6041 hypothesizes that the use of chemoradiation therapy before surgery will increase the proportion of patients who will have a resection with negative margins and will reduce the number of patients excluded from the analysis because of lack of compliance with the study guidelines. The study will also investigate the feasibility of using molecular techniques to assess tumor response to chemoradiation therapy. The investigators intend to enroll 85 patients in this phase of the trial. Although the study will not yield comparative results, it will catalyze the discourse on the impact of multimodal approaches to local, less invasive treatments for rectal cancer and, as the technology advances, may help guide future therapy for locally advanced disease (Table 13.1).

Conclusions and Recommendations for Future Trials

Relative to the standard radical operations, traditional approaches to local excision of rectal cancer were thought to result in narrower resection margins and retention of malignant cells in the mesorectum, potentiating recurrence of local disease. Conversely, local excision modalities seem to carry less perioperative clinical morbidity, avoiding the loss of gastrointestinal continuity, and in some studies decreasing operative time, postoperative analgesia requirements and length of stay. Although to date, there are no published prospective randomized trials comparing traditional transanal excision of rectal tumors with radical resection, there are solid clinical trial outcomes to support an increased role for the TEM approach in select cases. TEM increases transanal tumor visibility and accessibility, thus addressing previous criticism regarding poor adherence to oncological principles, while providing the aforementioned perioperative clinical benefits.

Given the tremendous potential of this technique particularly in patients diagnosed with early-stage disease and the recent advances in medical oncology, which have improved our ability to downstage tumors with neoadjuvant therapy, the need for future clinical trials comparing local resection with radical proctectomy is somewhat unclear. Perhaps we should, as suggested by the ongoing ACOSOG study, shift our focus toward the comparisons of various multimodal therapies to downstage rectal cancers, opening the door for the application of minimally invasive techniques under a broader range of clinical circumstances. Just as in the ACOSOG study, future trials should also consider the effect on quality of life in addition to oncological efficacy.

Table 13.1 American College of Surgeons Oncology Group Z6041 phase II trial of neoadjuvant chemoradiation therapy and local excision for uT2uN0 rectal cancer. *CRT* chemoradiation therapy, *LE* local excision. (Printed with permission of the American College of Surgeons Oncology Group)

ACOSOG: American College of Surgeons Oncology Group	**Z6041** Study Synopsis
Gastrointestinal Organ Site Committee	Study Chair: Julio Garcia-Aguilar, MD
TITLE	A Phase II Trial of Neoadjuvant Chemoradiation and Local Excision for uT2uN0 Rectal Cancer
SCHEMA	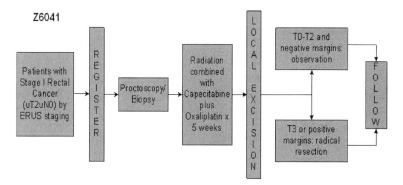
OBJECTIVES	**Primary Objective**
	To determine the rate of disease-free survival at 3 years in ultrasound-staged uT2uN0 rectal cancer patients treated with CRT followed by LE. Disease-free survival is defined as: no evidence of death, and no evidence of recurrence or distant metastasis on clinical, radiological, or ultrasound exam at the specified time.
	Secondary Objectives
	• To determine the rate of resectability with negative margins in ultrasound-staged uT2uN0 rectal cancer treated with neoadjuvant CRT followed by LE
	• To determine the procedure-specific morbidity and mortality following neoadjuvant CRT and LE
	• To determine the rate of pathologic complete response of the primary tumor to a CRT regimen including capecitabine plus oxaliplatin
	• To explore the impact of neoadjuvant CRT followed by LE on anorectal function and quality of life
	• To explore the feasibility of using molecular studies to assess surgical resection margins and tumor response to neoadjuvant CRT
	• To explore molecular markers associated with local tumor recurrence
STUDY DESIGN	This is a single arm, non-randomized, multi-center, phase II clinical trial evaluating the efficacy and safety of a multi-modality treatment consisting of high-dose external-beam radiation combined with capecitabine plus oxaliplatin, followed by local excision in patients with ultrasound-staged uT2uN0 rectal cancer.
	The primary endpoint of the study is disease-free survival. Suspected tumor recurrence within the surgical and/or radiation field should be documented histologically or cytologically. Pathological documentation of suspected distant metastasis is also recommended.

13 Clinical Trials

Table 13.1 (continued)

	Pathologic response will be determined by comparing tumor width and stage in the surgical specimen with the same parameters as determined by pre-CRT ERUS: • Pathologic Complete Response (pCR): no residual tumor. • Pathologic Progressive Disease (pPD): at least a 20% increase in tumor greatest diameter. • Pathologic Downstage (pDS): pathologic stage lower than ERUS stage.
	After completion of treatment patient will receive an initial post-surgical exam at 1 month after completion of surgery. Follow-up will consist of anal digital exam, proctoscopy and ERUS every 4 months for 3 years, and then every six months for the following 2 years. Quality of Life and anorectal function instruments (FISI/FIQL/FACT-C) will be administered 1 year (12 months) after surgery.
	In addition, patients will undergo colonoscopy 3 years (36 months) after surgery. The colonoscopy will be performed at physician discretion if polyps are found at any scheduled exams. Other diagnostic tests to detect or confirm tumor recurrence or distal metastasis may be performed if clinically indicated.
ACCRUAL GOAL	Z6041 is projected to accrue 85 eligible patients.
ELIGIBILITY CRITERIA	**Inclusion Criteria** 1. Patient must be at least 18 years of age. 2. Patient must have an ECOG/Zubrod status of ≤ 2. 3. Patient must have histologically confirmed invasive adenocarcinoma of the rectum. 4. Distal border of the patient's tumor must be within 8 cm from the anal verge as measured on rigid proctoscopic exam. 5. Patients with tumors fixed to adjacent structures on digital exam are NOT eligible. 6. Patient must have an uT2uN0 tumor, as confirmed by ERUS scan. Patients with uT1, uT3, or uT4 tumors are NOT eligible. Greatest diameter of tumor cannot exceed 4 cm. 7. Patients with positive perirectal nodes on ERUS examination are NOT eligible. 8. Patients with histologic evidence of metastatic invasion of inguinal lymph nodes are NOT eligible. 9. Patients with the following conditions are NOT allowed on study: • Metastatic disease or other primaries (patient must have had Chest X-ray/CT and Abdominal/Pelvic CT/MRI with IV contrast, as well as colonoscopy). • Previously documented history of Familial Adenomatous Polyposis • Previously documented history of Hereditary Non-Polyposis Colorectal Cancer diagnosed clinically (Amsterdam II criteria) or by genetic testing • History of Inflammatory Bowel Disease • History of prior radiation treatments to pelvis • Clinically significant peripheral sensory or motor neuropathy (defined as symptomatic weakness, paresthesia or sensory alteration described to be interfering with function, interfering with activities of daily living, disabling or life-threatening) • History of any clinically significant cardiac disease (i.e., Class 3-4 congestive heart failure, symptomatic coronary artery disease, uncontrolled arrhythmia, and/or myocardial infarction within the last 6 months) • History of uncontrolled seizures or clinically significant central nervous system disorders.

Table 13.1 (continued)

- History of psychiatric conditions or diminished mental capacity that could compromise the giving of informed consent, or interfere with study compliance

- History of allergy and/or hypersensitivity to Capecitabine and/or Oxaliplatin

- History of difficulty or inability to take or absorb oral medications

10. Patient must have adequate bone marrow, hepatic and renal function prior to registration:

- WBC $\geq$ 3000/mm3

- ANC > 1,500/mm3

- Hemoglobin > 9.5 mg/dl

- Platelet count $\geq$ 100,000/mm3

- Total bilirubin $\leq$ 3 mg/dl

- AST (SGOT) $\leq$ 2.0 times institutional upper limit of normal (ULN)

- ALT (SGPT) $\leq$ 2.0 times ULN

- Alkaline phosphatase $\leq$ 2.0 times ULN

- Creatinine clearance (CLcr) $\geq$ 50 ml/min by Cockroft-Gault Equation*:

*Cockcroft-Gault formula:

Male: Creatinine Clearance = (140 – age) x weight/(72 X serum creatinine)
Female: Creatinine Clearance = (140 – age) x weight/(72 X serum creatinine) x 0.85

11. Patients who have experienced a prior malignancy must have received potentially curative therapy for that malignancy, and must be cancer –free for at least five years from the date of initial diagnosis (Exceptions: patients treated for basal cell carcinoma, or carcinoma insitu of the cervix).

12. Baseline anorectal function must be measured and documented by the Fecal Incontinence Severity Index (FISI).

13. Patients of reproductive potential must agree to use an effective method of birth control when undergoing treatments with known or possible mutagenic or teratogenic effects. All female participants of childbearing potential must have a negative urine or serum pregnancy test within two weeks prior study registration.

14. Patient or the patient's legally acceptable representative must provide a signed and dated written informed consent prior to registration and any study-related procedures. NOTE: The signed and dated written consent form must be obtained from the patient prior to study registration or the initiation of any study-specific procedures.

15. Patient or the patient's legally acceptable representative must provide written authorization to allow the use and disclosure of their protected health information.* NOTE: This may be obtained in either the study-specific informed consent or in a separate authorization form and must be obtained from the patient prior to study registration or the initiation of any study-specific procedures.

SPECIMEN COLLECTION

In this study the following tissue samples will be submitted:

- A formalin-fixed biopsy sample taken from the tumor before radiation.

- Representative samples from the tumor and adjacent normal rectal wall. Paraffin blocks are strongly preferred; however, if the blocks are not available, histology slides are acceptable. Representative section of tumor tissue and normal rectal wall prepared during the transanal excision should be sent along with a copy of the finalized pathology report.

- Resection margins obtained from the edges of the tumor bed after removal of the surgical specimens.

References

1. Rothenberger DA, Wong WD. Abdominoperineal resection for adenocarcinoma of the low rectum. World J Surg, 1992. 16 (3): 478–85
2. Hughes ES, McDermott FT, Masterton JP, Polglase AL. Operative mortality following excision of the rectum. Br J Surg, 1980. 67 (1): 49–51
3. Williams NS, Johnston D. The quality of life after rectal excision for low rectal cancer. Br J Surg, 1983. 70 (8): 460–2
4. Karanjia ND, Schache DJ, Heald RJ. Function of the distal rectum after low anterior resection for carcinoma. Br J Surg, 1992. 79 (2): 114–6
5. Lee SJ, Park YS. Serial evaluation of anorectal function following low anterior resection of the rectum. Int J Colorectal Dis, 1998. 13 (5): 241
6. Bentrem DJ, Okabe S, Wong WD, Paty PB. T1 adenocarcinoma of the rectum: transanal excision or radical surgery? Ann Surg, 2005. 242 (4): 472–7
7. Endreseth BH. Transanal excision versus major surgery for T1 rectal cancer. Dis Colon Rectum, 2005. 48 (7): 1380–8
8. Mellgren, A, Sirivongs P, Rothenberger DA, Madoff RD, Garcia-Aguilar J. Is local excision adequate therapy for early rectal cancer? Dis Colon Rectum, 2000. 43 (8): 1064–71
9. Nascimbeni R, Nivatvongs S, Larson DR, Burgart LJ. Long-term survival after local excision for T1 carcinoma of the rectum. Dis Colon Rectum, 2004. 47 (11): 1773–9
10. Buess G, Theiss R, Pichlmaier H. [Transanal Endoscopic Microsurgery] *Leber Magen Darm,* 1985. 15 (6): 271–9
11. Burghardt J, Buess G. Transanal endoscopic microsurgery (TEM): a new technique and development during a time period of 20 years. Surg Technol Int, 2005:14:131–7
12. Russell AH, et al. Anal sphincter conservation for patients with adenocarcinoma of the distal rectum: long-term results of radiation therapy oncology group protocol 89-02. Int J Radiat Oncol Biol Phys, 2000. 46 (2):313–22
13. *NEW* Steele GD, et al. Sphincter-sparing treatment for distal recual adenocarcinoma. Ann Surg Oncol, 1999. 6 (5): 433–41
14. Winde G, Nottberg H, Keller R, Schmid KW, Bunte H. Surgical cure for early rectal carcinomas (T1). Transanal endoscopic microsurgery versus anterior resection. Dis Colon Rectum, 1996. 39 (9): 969–76
15. Lezoche E, Guerrieri M, Paganini AM, De Sanctis A. Transanal endoscopic versus total mesorectal laparoscopic resections of T2N0 low rectal cancers after neoadjuvant treatment. Surg Endosc, 2005. 19: 751–6
16. Lezoche E, Guerrieri M, De Sanctis A, Perretta S. Management of T2N0 rectal tumors: long-term randomized study comparing transanal endoscopic microsurgery versus laparoscopic resections. Last on line access 11/28/2006 http://www.ssat.com/cgi-bin/abstracts/06ddw/SSAT_DDW06_80.cgi
17. Cataldo PA, O'Brien S, Osler T. Transanal endoscopic microsurgery: a prospective evaluation of functional results. Dis Colon Rectum, 2005. 48 (7): 1366–71
18. National Cancer Institute website. Last access 12/19/2006 http://www.cancer.gov/search/ViewClinicalTrials.aspx
19. National Institutes of Health website. Last access 11/29/2006 http://www.clinicaltrials.gov
20. Dana Farber Cancer Institute. Last access 12/19/2006 http://www.danafarber.org/can/clinical
21. Memorial-Sloan Kettering Cancer Center. Last access 12/19/2006 http://www.mskcc.org/mskcc/html/5707.cfm
22. MD Anderson Cancer Center. Last access 11/29/2006 http://www.mdanderson.org/patients_public/clinical_trials

Chapter 14
Future Directions

Mark Choh and Theodore J. Saclarides

Introduction

Since transanal endoscopic microsurgery (TEM) was introduced in the mid-1980s, it has been well established that the technique is a safe and effective method to excise adenomas of the rectum. It is also clear that rectal carcinomas can adequately be resected using TEM techniques if appropriate patient selection criteria are employed. Many of these lesions would have previously required a laparotomy for removal. In addition, removal of other lesions such as carcinoids, rectal schwannomas, and rectal endometriosis has been described [1–4]. Currently, the spectrum of uses for TEM is mainly limited to those just mentioned. With respect to extended applications, all that is required is creative thinking.

Currently, there are only scattered mentions in the literature reporting the use of TEM for conditions other than the excision of rectal tumors. Salm et al. [5] retrospectively reviewed 1,900 TEM-assisted procedures performed in Germany at 57 centers—of these, only 2.9% were performed for indications other than adenomas or carcinomas. However, surgeons are beginning to realize its potential as a minimal-access alternative to rectal abnormalities. Among those procedures being described are posterior transrectal rectopexy for rectal prolapse, repair of rectovaginal fistulas, ablation or lysis of fibrotic or anastomotic rectal strictures, and endorectal advancement flaps for high anorectal fistulas. While TEM should not be considered the standard of care for any of the abovementioned conditions, when proper patient selection criteria are used, it can become a useful adjunct for the treatment of rectal disease.

TEM has continued to build momentum since its introduction. The literature now clearly supports its use to resect large adenomas that cannot be removed endoscopically, and the number of TEM centers in the USA and around the world is growing. In addition, newer operative techniques, such as the use of ultracision and laser technology, and improvement in suture techniques have facilitated the use of TEM as an adjunct to the treatment of rectal abnormalities [6–8]. The initial overhead cost for the TEM equipment, however, may be prohibitive for some centers, and concerns about reimbursement may cause hesitation amongst prospective surgeons.

M. Choh (✉)
Rush Medical College, Rush University Medical Center, Chicago, IL, USA

P.A. Cataldo, G.F. Buess (eds.), *Transanal Endoscopic Microsurgery*,
DOI 10.1007/978-0-387-76397-2_14, © Springer Science + Business Media, LLC 2009

Rectal Prolapse

Rectal prolapse, or procidentia, occurs when a full-thickness portion of the rectum protrudes beyond the anal canal. Lack of posterior rectal fixation to the sacrum and laxity of the mesorectum results in redundancy of the rectosigmoid colon, enabling the bowel to prolapse. The disease primarily affects women, with 80–90% of cases being reported in women [9]. It is also a disease of the elderly, with an increasing incidence starting during the sixth decade. Prolapse causes a great deal of morbidity and lifestyle problems for those whom are affected by it, as debilitating symptoms such as fecal incontinence and severe constipation are common.

Traditional methods of treatment are divided into transabdominal and perineal operations. The transabdominal operations include suture or prosthetic mesh rectopexy, the Ripstein anterior sling, or a formal low anterior resection. These procedures may be performed laparoscopically. Perineal procedures, such as the Delorme procedure and the Altemeier perineal rectosigmoidectomy, are preferred in higher-risk patients because they obviate the need for laparotomy. TEM has been used to perform a posterior, transrectal rectopexy for prolapse; however, its use has been somewhat limited in this regard.

The patient is given general anesthesia and is then placed in the lithotomy position. After setup of the TEM apparatus, the rectoscope is inserted and carbon dioxide is insufflated. A transverse full-thickness incision is made in the posterior rectal wall and this is carried down through the perirectal fat using sharp dissection or electrocautery. This releases the redundant rectum, which is then pushed cephalad. In addition, by dissecting in this space, one exposes the presacral fascia. The released rectum is then brought superiorly and anchored (using the full thickness of the rectal wall to the presacral tissue) with interrupted suture using techniques described earlier. The rectal incision is then closed transversely.

Rectovaginal Fistula/Extrasphincteric Fistula-In-Ano

Rectovaginal fistulas may cause a great deal of morbidity and distress. They most commonly result from perineal injuries sustained during childbirth; however, radiation therapy for rectal or gynecologic tumors, inflammatory conditions such as Crohn's disease, and infectious causes are also commonly implicated. Most rectovaginal fistulas occur in the lower third of the rectum and can be repaired via traditional transanal, transvaginal, or transperineal techniques. High rectovaginal fistulas, however, occur between the middle and upper third of the rectum and the posterior wall of the vagina, and may require a laparotomy for repair. Iatrogenic fistulas may occur during stapled colorectal anastomoses following proctectomy for rectal cancer. In these instances, the vagina is inadvertently included in the staple line, resulting in a fistula. Most of these fistulas are too high to be repaired with conventional transanal or transvaginal techniques. Posterior approaches to the rectum using paracoccygeal incisions may not be able to reach the fistula. Furthermore, nonhealing of the posterior rectotomy used to approach the fistula may occur, leading to a sacral fistula in 20% of patients. The final option potentially available for these patients is a laparotomy, completion proctectomy with coloanal anastomosis with or without construction of a colonic reservoir. This is a technically demanding operation in a pelvis previously operated on and perhaps also exposed to radiation in some instances. Significant fibrosis can be expected, causing lengthy surgery and bleeding. A TEM-assisted approach to stapler-induced fistulas is therefore an approach with attractive advantages.

Patient selection is critical in choosing which patients may benefit from a TEM-assisted repair. Older patients with multiple medical problems who present a prohibitive operative risk for transabdominal repair via laparotomy may be potential candidates. Crohn's disease patients with high fistulas and multiple prior laparotomies may also be considered for TEM repair. Patients with high rectovaginal fistulas occurring as a result of previous pelvic irradiation may be candidates as the radiation-induced changes in the pelvis and surgical adhesions may make dissection of the rectovaginal septum extremely difficult. In these latter instances, however, the irradiated rectum may not accommodate the 40-mm TEM rectoscope because of the fibrotic changes that accompany exposure to radiation. The same may be true for Crohn's disease. Iatrogenic rectovaginal fistulas following stapled colorectal anastomoses may also be problematic for TEM repair. In these instances, the diminished capacity of the rectum in addition to its loss of compliance if radiation therapy was given may hinder placement of the TEM rectoscope. Experience is limited and anecdotal: however, conceptually there is no reason not to try TEM repair for complicated rectovaginal fistulas.

Extrasphincteric fistulas to the buttocks or perineum may originate from the rectal wall high above the dentate line. Causes include inflammatory bowel disease, trauma, or foreign objects. Fistulotomy is unacceptable because of potential sphincter damage, and flap repair has been a favored approach. Alternatives include the use of fibrin glue and collagen plugs; however, results have been mixed. Flap construction may be difficult if the primary opening is located several centimeters above the anal canal; hence, the potential utility for TEM technology.

Modification of the traditional transanal advancement flap repair of low rectovaginal fistulas may be applied to TEM-assisted repair of more proximal rectovaginal fistulas and extrasphincteric fistulas. Since the procedure is performed anteriorly for vaginal fistulas, the patient is placed in the prone position after the induction of general anesthesia. The TEM rectoscope is inserted and the fistula tract is visualized. In cases of rectovaginal fistulas, loss of CO_2 through the vagina can be avoided by occlusion of the vagina with a balloon. One raises a flap consisting of mucosa, submucosa, and circular muscle, extending cephalad at least 4 cm. The flap must have a broad base to ensure an adequate blood supply to the apex. The distal portion of the flap containing the fistula tract is excised, and the remaining tract is curettaged. The rectovaginal septum is closed longitudinally. The rectal flap is then advanced caudally and sutured in place, covering the closure of the septum.

Anastomotic Stricture

Unfortunately, strictures after stapled anastomosis during low anterior resection do not happen infrequently—rates up to 30% have been reported. Risk factors include advanced patient age, exposure to radiation, inflammatory bowel disease, and diversion of the fecal stream. Many are asymptomatic and are only be diagnosed on proctoscopy or endoscopy; when symptomatic, patients present with symptoms or partial or complete colonic obstruction. Most can be treated conservatively with balloon or bougie dilation or cautery using thermal or laser energy under rigid or flexible endoscopic guidance. In rare cases, operative resection is needed.

However, TEM-assisted therapy can be an option to treat anastomotic strictures in certain patients. Kato et al. [8] described the treatment of a short-segment 0.8-cm-diameter anastomotic stricture that recurred after bougie and balloon dilatation. A contact Nd:YAG laser system was used to release the stricture, and the patient was asymptomatic as of 9 months after the operation. In addition, it may be used to treat strictures by using electrocautery or by operative sleeve resection. The additional length provided by the TEM rectoscope may allow transanal treatment of more proximal strictures that may have required a transabdominal approach. Also, the stereoscopic optics of TEM combined with the constant insufflation will facilitate more precise operative treatment of more distally located strictures compared with conventional transanal surgery.

Extended Applications for Cancer Patients

While TEM can provide acceptable cure rates for patients with early, superficial cancers, most would argue that local excision of any form should not be performed for pT2 and pT3 cancers. Nodal metastases are not addressed and local recurrence rates of 30 and 50%, respectively, can be expected. Multimodality therapy with radiation therapy and chemotherapy may be used as adjuncts to local excision. The driving force behind this concept is the knowledge that chemoradiation therapy will significantly shrink large lesions down to small ulcers or plaques, fewer metastatic lymph nodes are found following radical surgery, and complete histologic response rates of up to 30% may be found. Local excision of the original tumor site has been proposed as a means of deciding whether additional surgery is needed. Namely, if no residual disease is found at the original site, then one may assume that nodal disease may have been successfully ablated as well. Obviously, further work within these areas must be done to determine if this logic is sound and whether acceptable cure rates can be obtained.

The question arises whether TEM should be performed before or after radiation therapy and chemotherapy. If TEM is performed first, then the exact depth of penetration by the tumor will be known; if the lesion is a pT2 or pT3 tumor, adjuvant therapy is indicated. If TEM is performed after radiation therapy and chemotherapy, one can use the intramural tumor response to multimodality therapy to estimate the likelihood of persistent nodal disease. A complete histologic response may be an indicator that the nodal metastases have been treated. It is not known how extensive the local excision should be. That is, should the size of the resected specimen match the tumor size before treatment, or should it be tailored according to its response to treatment?

Another potential application of TEM is the sampling of sentinel lymph nodes. Research needs to establish the feasibility of accessing the sentinel nodes transanally via a posterior rectotomy. It is conceivable that the location of these nodes may be influenced by gender, distance of the tumor from the anal canal, anterior–posterior orientation of the lesion within the rectum, and whether radiation therapy has been given.

Coding

TEM does not have its own procedural code. Options include 45170—the conventional code for transanal excision of a neoplasm, 45123—partial proctectomy without anastomosis, and 45999—unlisted procedure, rectum. The first option, namely, transanal

14 Future Directions

Table 14.1 Reimbursement rates (in dollars) for third parties in Region 16, Illinois, USA

	Code 45123	Code 45170
Medicare	1,066.57	761.04
Aetna	1,523.09	1,100.27
Blue Cross	1,487.00	1,061.00
Cigna	1,356.04	979.59
Great West	1,446.86	896.42
Humana	1,368.91	969.71

excision, does not reimburse at a rate that reflects the advanced training required to master TEM techniques, the demanding nature of TEM, and the high cost of the equipment. Code 45123 reimburses at a higher rate. Code 45999 may allow one to bill at an even higher rate but creates a potential cumbersome paper trail. Table 14.1 shows reimbursement rates by code for certain third-party payers in Region 16, Illinois, USA.

Conclusions

Virtually all of the published literature on TEM has dealt with excising adenomas and selected cancers. It is a safe technique for addressing these lesions. Once TEM has been mastered, virtually any pathologic problem involving the rectum can be tackled with the TEM instrumentation. All that is required is innovative thinking. It may even have a role in natural orifice surgery. This chapter has attempted to stimulate thinking along these lines.

References

1. Saclarides TJ. Transanal endoscopic microsurgery: a single surgeon's Experience. Archives of Surgery 133(6): 595–8; discussion 598–9, 1998.
2. Guillem JG, Chessin DB, Jeong SY, Kim W, Fogarty JM. Contemporary applications of transanal endoscopic microsurgery: technical innovations and limitations. Clinical Colorectal Cancer 5(4): 268–73, 2005.
3. Kakizoe S, Kuwahara S, Kakizoe K, Kakizoe H, Kakizoe Y, Kakizoe T, Yamamoto O, Kakizoe S. Local excision of benign rectal schwannoma using rectal expander-assisted transanal endoscopic microsurgery. Gastrointestinal Endoscopy 48(1): 90–2, 1998.
4. Kilgus M, Schöb O, Largiadèr F. Rectal endometriosis: transanal endoscopic microsurgery or laparoscopic resection? European Journal of Surgery 164(3): 231–2, 1998.
5. Salm R, Lampe H, Bustos A, Matern U. Experience with TEM in Germany. Endoscopic Surgery & Allied Technologies 2(5):251–4, 1994.
6. Ayodeji ID, Hop WC, Tetteroo GW, Bonjer HJ, deGraaf EJ. Ultracision harmonic scalpel and multifunctional tem400 instrument complement in transanal endoscopic microsurgery: a prospective study. Surgical Endoscopy 18(12): 1730–7, 2004.
7. Lirici MM, DiPaola M, Ponzano C, Hüscher CG. Combining ultrasonic dissection and the Storz operation rectoscope. Surgical Endoscopy 17(8): 1292–7, 2003.
8. Kato K, Saito T, Matsuda M, Imai M, Kasai S, Mito M. Successful treatment of a rectal anastomotic stenosis by transanal endoscopic microsurgery (TEM) using the contact Nd:YAG laser" Surgical Endoscopy 11(5): 485–7, 1997.
9. Madiba TE, Baig MK, Wexner SD. Surgical management of rectal prolapse. Archives of Surgery 140(1): 63–73, 2005.

Index

A

Abdominoperineal resection (APR), 117–118, 121
Adaptable laparoscopic instruments, 20–21, 20*f*, 27, 36
Adenomas
  benign rectal, 87–95, 88*t*–89*t*, 91*t*–94*t*
  full-thickness excision, 47
  indications, 1–4
  large, 41–42
  partial-thickness excision, 41–42
  rectal, 47
Advanced surgical techniques, 59–73
Anal condyloma, 27
Anal incontinence, 79–80
Anal stenosis, 27
Anal verge to peritoneal reflection,
         measurements, 3*t*
Anastomotic rectal strictures, 135, 137–138
Anesthesia, 22, 36
  full-thickness excision, 50
  partial-thickness excision, 42
Anovaginal fistula, 41, 45
Anovaginal septum, 31–32
Antibiotics, 9–10, 42
APR, *see* Abdominoperineal resection (APR)
Articulated stabilizing arm, 13, 14*f*, 22, 36
Atlas, 50

B

Biopsy, 48*f*
Bleeding, 7, 52, 77–78
Bone scintigraphy, 48
Bowel preparation, 9–10
Bowen's disease, 27

C

Carcinoma, 47
Cardiopulmonary complications, 81
Catheterization, 10
Chemoradiation therapy, 109–114, 126, 130*t*–132*t*
Chemoradiotherapy, 53, 56
Chemotherapy, 49
Chest X-ray, 48

Clinical trials
  chemoradiation therapy, 126, 130*t*–132*t*
  conclusions, recommendations, 129
  LAR, 125
  local excision, 126–127, 127*f*
  National Cancer Database, 127
  standardized neoadjuvant therapy regimen, 129
  TAE, 125
  TEM, 127–129
  TME, 125
Clip applier, 15, 18–19, 18*f*
CO_2, 14, 15*f*, 22, 36
Coding, 138–139
Colonoscopy, 48, 61
Complications, 7–8
  anal incontinence, 79–80
  bleeding, 77–78
  cardiopulmonary, 81
  conversion to laparotomy, 78–79
  dehiscence, 78
  extended full-thickness resection, 66
  fever, 81
  morbidity, 75–76
  mortality, 75–76
  partial-thickness excision, 45
  peritoneal entry, 77
  positioning, 81
  rare, 81
  rectal stenosis, 81
  rectovaginal fistula, 80–81
  urinary, 79
  See also Perioperative complications
Computed tomography (CT) scan, 48, 49, 61
Consent, 7–8
Contraindications, 3
CT scan, *see* Computed tomography (CT) scan

D

Debulking, 8–9
Deep venous thrombosis prophylaxis, 10
Dehiscence, 78
Denonvillier's fascia, 31

142 Index

Doxycycline, 113
DVD, 22

E
EBVS, *see* Electrothermal bipolar vessel sealing
  (EBVS)
Electric knife (electrocautery)
  equipment, 15–17, 18*f*, 24–25, 31, 36
  partial-thickness excision, 43, 43*f*
  pelvic anatomic considerations, 31
  set-up, operative, 36
  traditional techniques, 85
Electrothermal bipolar vessel sealing (EBVS), 50, 52
Endorectal advancement flaps, 135
Endorectal ultrasound, 48
Endoscopic biopsies, 48
Endoscopic piecemeal excision, 86
Endoscopy, 47
Epinephrine
  advanced procedures, 64, 67–68, 69–71
  complications, 78
  equipment, 18, 22
  partial-thickness excision, 43
  set-up, operative, 36
Equipment
  adaptable laparoscopic instruments, 20–21
  articulated stabilizing arm, 13, 14*f*, 15*f*, 22, 36
  Atlas, 50
  clip applier, 15, 18–19, 18*f*
  CO$_2$, 14, 15*f*, 22, 36
  description, 13
  EBVS, 50
  electric knife (electrocautery), 15–17, 18*f*, 24–25,
    31, 36
  faceplates, 14, 15*f*, 16*f*, 22, 36, 61
  forceps, 15, 17, 18*f*
  full-thickness excision, 50
  harmonic scalpel, 20, 20*f*, 31, 36, 50
  insufflator, 14, 16*f*, 19, 19*f*, 22–23, 23*f*, 36, 50
  irrigation reservoir, 19*f*
  laparoscope, 61, 63, 69
  laparoscopic camera, 15, 19*f*
  LigaSure, 20–21, 20*f*, 50
  long instruments, 15–19, 18*f*
  multidimensional instrument, 50
  needle holder, 15, 18, 18*f*
  obturator, 14, 14*f*
  optics, 15, 17*f*
  printer, 19*f*
  proctoscope, 13–15, 14*f*, 15*f*, 36, 61
  rectoscope, 50
  retractable needle, 15, 18, 18*f*
  Richard Wolf Company, 50, 61
  scissors, 15, 17, 18*f*
  suction probe, 15, 17–18, 18*f*
  tattooing, 18
  TEM cart, 19*f*, 22
  TEM pump, 19*f*

Tyco Healthcare, 50
VHS, slide printer, 19*f*
video monitor, 15, 17*f*, 19, 19*f*, 24
See also Set-up, operative
Extended full-thickness resection
  complications, 66
  indications, 62
  patient position, 63*f*, 64*f*
  perirectal tissue, 65*f*
  procedure, 63–66, 63*f*, 64*f*
  room preparation, 62–63
Extraluminal techniques
  Kraske, 86–87
  York–Mason, 87
Extraperitoneal rectum, 32–33, 32*f*
Extrarectal anatomy, 30–32, 31*f*
Extrasphincteric fistula-in-ano, 136–137

F
Faceplates, 14, 15*f*, 16*f*, 22, 36, 61
Fansler retractor, 85
Fecal diversion, 113
Fever, 81
Fibrotic rectal strictures, 135
Fistula
  anovaginal, 41, 45
  perioperative complications, 52–53
  rectovaginal, 42
Flexible endoscopes, 72–73, 73*f*
Flexible sigmoidoscopy, 113
Forceps, 15, 17, 18*f*
Formal celiotomy, 7
Full-thickness excision
  adenoma, rectal, 47
  anesthesia, 50
  Atlas, 50
  carcinomas, rectal, 47
  chemoradiotherapy, 53, 56
  chemotherapy, 49
  EBVS, 50
  harmonic scalpel, 50
  indications, 47
  informed consent, 49–50
  insufflator, 50
  lesions, T2, 49
  lesions, T3, 49
  LigaSure, 50
  lymphatic sampling, 55–56
  mucosectomy, 51, 51*f*
  multidimensional instrument, 50
  neoadjuvant therapy, 49
  neoplasia, 53
  partial rectal wall excision, 51, 51*f*
  patient preparation, 49
  perioperative complications
    bleeding, 52
    fistula, 52–53
    harmonic scalpel, 52

incontinence, 53
intraperitoneal entry, 52
LigaSure, 52
suture line disruption, 53
post-neoadjuvant-therapy staging
  endoscopy, 49
  radiochemotherapy, 49
  transanal ultrasound, 48
preoperative staging
  biopsy, 48*f*
  bone scintigraphy, 48
  chest X-ray, 48
  colonoscopy, total, 48
  CT scan, 48, 49
  endorectal ultrasound, 48
  endoscopic biopsies, 48
  macrobiopsy, 48
  metastasis, 48
  MRI, 48–49
  rectal cancer, 48*f*
  rectal wall penetration, 48
  rectoscopy, rigid, 48
  regional lymph nodes, 48
  transanal endosonography, 48
radiotherapy, 49, 54–55
rectal cancer, 54–56
rectoscope, 50
resection margins, 53, 54*f*
Stockholm randomized trials, 55
timing, 54–55
Tyco Healthcare, 50
Full-thickness local excision
  abdominopelvic CT scan, 113
  chemoradiation therapy, 109–114
  conclusion, 114
  doxycycline, 113
  fecal diversion, 113
  flexible sigmoidoscopy, 113
  follow-up, 113
  high-dose radiation therapy, 109–112
  history, 110–111
  loop ileostomy, 113
  morbidity, 113
  neoadjuvant therapy, 109–113
  outcomes, 111
  patient selection, 111–112, 111*f*
  permanent stoma, 110
  postoperative issues, 113
  radical proctectomy, 110
  radical resection, 110
  secondary goals, 109
  technical issues, 112–113
  three-tesla MRI scan, 113
  three-tesla PET scan, 113
  transverse loop colostomy, 113
Full-thickness resection, 7, 33
Future directions
  anastomotic rectal strictures, 135, 137–138

cancer patients, 138
coding, 138–139
endorectal advancement flaps, 135
extrasphincteric fistula-in-ano, 136–137
fibrotic rectal strictures, 135
high anorectal fistulas, 135
patient selection, 137
posterior transrectal rectopexy, rectal
    prolapse, 135
procidentia, 136
rectal prolapse, 136
rectovaginal fistula, 135, 136
reimbursement rates, 138–139, 139*t*

G
Gauges and regulating buttons, 24*f*

H
Harmonic scalpel, 20, 20*f*, 31, 36, 50, 52
Heparin, 10
High anorectal fistulas, 135
High-dose radiation therapy, 109–112

I
Incontinence, 7, 53
Indications
  adenoma, 1
  anal verge to peritoneal reflection, 3*t*
  contraindications, 3
  by disease process, 2*t*
  extended full-thickness resection, 62
  full-thickness excision, 47
  intraperitoneal entry, 3
  lesions, bulky, 3
  NOTES, 4
  partial-thickness excision, 41–42
  rectal polyps, 1–3
  resection, 1–2
  sleeve resection, 66
  strictures, 3
  TEM limitations, 3–4
  transrectal fistula repair, 68–69
Informed consent, 49–50
Insufflator, 14, 16*f*, 19, 19*f*, 23, 23*f*, 62
Intraluminal suturing, 37
Intraperitoneal entry, 3, 52
Irrigation reservoir, 19*f*

K
Kraske technique, 86–87

L
Laparoscopic camera, 15, 19*f*
Laparotomy, conversion to, 75, 76
Large-volume rectal resections, 28
LAR, *see* Low anterior resection (LAR)

Leaks, 14, 22, 24–25
Lesions
    bulky, 3
    evaluation, 8
    partial-thickness excision, 41
    preparation, 8–9
    T1, 49, 55, 103, 119–123, 127, 128
    T2, 8, 49, 98, 118–123
    T3, 8, 49, 54, 119, 122
    ultrasound, 8
    upper, 7–8
Lidocaine, 43, 43*f*, 78
LigaSure, 20–21, 20*f*, 31, 50, 52
Local excision, 126–127, 127*t*
Lone Star retractor, 85
Long instruments, 15–19, 18*f*
Loop ileostomy, 113
Low anterior resection (LAR), 117, 125
Luminal stenosis, 29–30
Lymphatic sampling, 55–56
Lymph nodes, regional, 48

M
Macrobiopsy, 48
Magnetic resonance imaging (MRI), 48–49
Martin arm, *see* Articulated stabilizing arm
Mesorectum, 30–31, 31*f*
Metastasis, 48
Morbidity, 75–76, 113
Mortality, 75–76
MRI, *see* Magnetic resonance imaging (MRI)
Mucosectomy, 51, 51*f*
Multidimensional instrument, 50

N
National Cancer Database, 127
Natural orifice transluminal endoscopic surgery
        (NOTES), 4, 72–73
Needle holder, 15, 18, 18*f*
Neoadjuvant therapy
    chemotherapy, 49
    full-thickness local excision, 109–114
    lesions, T2, 49
    lesions, T3, 49
    radiotherapy, 49, 54–55
    Stockholm randomized trials, 55
    timing, 54–55
Neoplasia, 53
NOTES, *see* Natural orifice transluminal
        endoscopic surgery (NOTES)

O
Obturator, 14, 14*f*
Oncologic outcomes
    APR, 117–118, 121
    conclusions, 123

historical background, 118
introduction, 117–118
LAR, 117
preoperative assessment, 119
radiotherapy, 121*t*, 122*t*
transanal endoscopic microsurgery,
        120, 122, 122*t*
transanal local excision, 119–121, 121*t*
Operating table, 21, 21*f*, 36
Optics, 15, 17*f*

P
Partial rectal wall excision, 51, 51*f*
Partial-thickness excision
    adenomas, large, 41–42
    anesthetic, 42
    anovaginal fistula, 41, 45
    antibiotics, 42
    complications, 45
    electric knife (electrocautery), 43, 43*f*
    epinephrine, 43
    indications, 41–42
    lidocaine, 43, 43*f*
    malignant lesions, 41
    operative technique, 42–44
    polyps, 41, 43*f*, 44*f*
    positioning patient, 42
    postoperative care, 44–45
    preoperative preparation, 42
    rectovaginal fistula, 42
    split-leg table attachments, 42
    submucosal excision, 41, 42*f*
    sutures, 42
    venous thromboembolism prophylaxis, 42
Patient positioning, *see* Positioning patient
Patient preparation, 49, 62
Patient selection, 38, 59–60, 111–112, 111*f*
Pelvic anatomic considerations
    anal condyloma, 27
    anal stenosis, 27
    anovaginal septum, 31
    Bowen's disease, 27
    defecatory function, 28
    Denonvillier's fascia, 31
    electric knife (electrocautery), 31
    extraperitoneal rectum, 32–33, 32*f*
    extrarectal anatomy, 30–32, 31*f*
    full-thickness resection, 33
    harmonic scalpel, 31
    large-volume rectal resections, 28
    LigaSure, 31
    luminal stenosis, 29–30
    mesorectum, 30–31, 31*f*
    peritoneal barrier, 33
    peritoneal envelope, 33
    peritoneal reflections, 32–33, 32*f*
    rectal access, 27–28
    rectal ampulla, 28, 30*f*

Index 145

rectosigmoid junction, 28–29, 29*f*
rectovaginal fistula, 30
rectum, 28–30, 29*f*, 30*f*
sentinal node technology, 31
sphincteric defects, 27–28
squamous cell cancer, 27
valves of Houston, 28, 29*f*
Perioperative complications
bleeding, 52
fistula, 52–53
full-thickness excision, 52–53
harmonic scalpel, 52
incontinence, 53
intraperitoneal entry, 52
LigaSure, 52
suture line disruption, 53
See also Complications
Perirectal tissue, 65*f*
Peritoneal
barrier, 33
entry, 77
envelope, 33
reflections, 32–33, 32*f*
Permanent stoma, 110
Pneumorectum, 23
Polyps, 41, 43*f*, 44*f*
Positioning patient, 8, 21–22, 36–39
complications, 81
extended full-thickness resection, 63*f*, 64*f*
partial-thickness excision, 42
Posterior transrectal rectopexy, rectal prolapse, 135
Post-neoadjuvant-therapy staging
endoscopy, 49
full-thickness excision, 49
radiochemotherapy, 49
Postoperative care, 44–45, 113
Pratt bivalve retractor, 85
Preoperative preparation
antibiotics, 10
bowel preparation, 9–10
cleaning, 9
enema, 9
consent, 7–8
bleeding, 7
complications, 7–8
formal celiotomy, 7
full-thickness resection, 7
incontinence, 7
resection, 7
risk factors, 7–8, 10
upper rectal lesion, 7–8
debulking, 8–9
deep venous thrombosis prophylaxis, heparin, 10
lesions
evaluation, 8
preparation, 8–9
T2, 8

T3, 8
ultrasound, 8
partial-thickness excision, 42
tattooing, 8–9
urinary retention, 10
catheterization, 10
venous thromboembolism, 10
Preoperative staging
biopsy, 48*f*
bone scintigraphy, 48
chest X-ray, 48
colonoscopy, total, 48
CT, 48–49
endorectal ultrasound, 48
endoscopic biopsies, 48
macrobiopsy, 48
metastasis, 48
MRI, 48, 49
rectal wall penetration, 48
rectoscopy, rigid, 48
regional lymph nodes, 48
transanal endosonography, 48
Preoperative workup, 61
Printer, 19*f*
Procidentia, 136
Proctoscope, 13, 14*f*, 36, 61

R
Radical proctectomy, 110
Radical resection, 110
Radiochemotherapy, 49
Radiotherapy, 49, 54–55, 121*t*, 122*t*
Rectal
access, 27–28
adenoma, 47
ampulla, 28, 30*f*
benign adenoma, 87–95, 88*t*–89*t*, 91*t*–94*t*
cancer, 1–4, 48*f*, 54–56, 95–105, 96*t*–97*t*
fistulae, 60
lesion, upper, 7–8
polyps, 1–3
prolapse, 136
stenosis, 81
ultrasound, 61
wall penetration, 48
Rectoscope, 50
Rectoscopy, 48
Rectosigmoid junction, 28–29, 29*f*
Rectovaginal fistula, 32, 42, 80–81, 136–137
Rectum, 28–30, 29*f*, 30*f*
Reimbursement rates, 138–139, 139*t*
Resection margins, 53, 54*f*
Retractable needle, 15–16, 18, 18*f*
Richard Wolf Company, 50, 61
Risk factors, 7–8, 10

S

Sawyer retractor, 85
Scheduling TEM procedures, 39
Scissors, 15, 17, 18*f*
Sentinal node technology, 31
Set-up, operative
  CO_2, 36
  DVD, 22
  gauges, regulating buttons, 23*f*
  leaks, 14, 22, 23–24
  operating table, 21–23, 21*f*, 36
  pneumorectum, 23–24
  split-leg table attachments, 36, 42
  stirrups, 21–22
  sutures, 22
  troubleshooting, 23–25
  videotape, 22
  See also Equipment
ShapeLock device, 72–73, 73*f*
Sleeve resection
  advanced techniques, 60
  anastomotic rectal strictures, 137–138
  caudal retraction, 67, 67*f*
  complications, 68
  indications, 66
  procedure, 67–68
  room preparation, 66
  stay sutures, 67, 67*f*
Sphincteric defects, 27–28
Split-leg table attachments, 36, 42
Squamous cell cancer, 27
Stirrups, 21
Stockholm randomized trials, 55
Submucosal excision, 41, 44*f*
Suction probe, 15, 17–18, 18*f*
Surgeon selection, 61
Suture line disruption, 53
Sutures, 4, 7, 28
  intraluminal suturing, 37
  long instruments, 18–19
  partial-thickness excision, 44
  set-up, operative, 22

T

TAE, *see* Transanal excision (TAE)
Tattooing, 8–10, 18, 53, 67–68
TEM, *see* Transanal endoscopic microsurgery
  (TEM)
TEM *vs* TAE, 87–90, 103–104, 103*t*
Three-tesla MRI scan, 113
Three-tesla PET scan, 113
TME, *see* Total mesorectal excision (TME)
Total mesorectal excision (TME), 125
Traditional techniques
  comparison studies, 103–104, 103*t*
  electric knife (electrocautery), 85
  endoscopic piecemeal excision, 86
  extraluminal techniques, 86–87

Fansler retractor, 85
  Kraske, 86–87
  Lone Star retractor, 85
  Pratt bivalve retractor, 85
  Sawyer retractor, 85
  TAE results, 87–90, 95–98, 88*t*–89*t*
  TEM results, 90–95, 91*t*–94*t*
  TEM *vs* TAE, 87–90, 103–105, 103*t*
  York–Mason, 87
Training, 17*f*, 22, 35
  courses, 37
  early experience, 38
  learning curve, 39
  nurses, 37
  sets, 36
Transanal endoscopic microsurgery (TEM)
  cart, 19*f*, 22
  clinical trials, 127–129
  contraindications, 3
  description, 35
  equipment, 13–21, 36–37
  indications, 1–4
  limitations, 3–4
  oncologic outcomes, 122–123, 122*t*
  patient selection, 38
  pump, 19*f*
  rectal adenoma, benign, 90–95, 91*t*–94*t*
  scheduling procedures, 37
Transanal endosonography, 48
Transanal excision (TAE)
  clinical trials, 128–129
  oncologic outcomes, 119–121, 121*t*
  results, rectal cancer, 95–98, 96*t*–97*t*
  traditional techniques, 85–86, 87–90,
    88*t*–89*t*
Transanal intraabdominal endoscopic
    surgery, 60–61
Transanal ultrasound, 49
Transrectal fistula repair
  complications, 71–72
  indications, 68–69
  patient preparation, 69
  procedure, 69–71, 69*t*, 70*f*, 71*f*, 72*f*
  room preparation, 69
Transverse loop colostomy, 113
Troubleshooting, 23–25
Tyco Healthcare, 50

U

Ultrasound
  endorectal, 48
  lesions, 8
  rectal, 61
  transanal, 49
Upper rectal lesion, 7–8
Urinary complications, 79
Urinary retention, 10

Index 147

V
Valves of Houston, 28, 29*f*
Venous thromboembolism, 10
Venous thromboembolism prophylaxis, 42
VHS and slide printer, 19*f*

Video monitor, 15, 17*f*, 19, 19*f*, 24
Videotape, 22

Y
York–Mason technique, 87

Printed in the United States of America

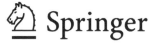

© Springer Science+Business Media, LLC 2009

This electronic component package is protected by federal copyright law and international treaty. If you wish to return this book and the electronic component package to Springer Science+Business Media, LLC, do not open the disc envelope or remove it from the book. Springer Science+Business Media, LLC, will not accept any returns if the package has been opened and/or separated from the book. The copyright holder retains title to and ownership of the package. U.S. copyright law prohibits you from making any copy of the entire electronic component package for any reason without the written permission of Springer Science+Business Media, LLC, except that you may download and copy the files from the electronic component package for your own research, teaching, and personal communications use. Commercial use without the written consent of Springer Science+Business Media, LLC, is strictly prohibited. Springer Science+Business Media, LLC, or its designee has the right to audit your computer and electronic components usage to determine whether any unauthorized copies of this package have been made.

Springer Science+Business Media, LLC, or the author(s) makes no warranty or representation, either express or implied, with respect to this electronic component package or book, including their quality, merchantability, or fitness for a particular purpose. In no event will Springer Science+Business Media, LLC, or the author(s) be liable for direct, indirect, special, incidental, or consequential damages arising out of the use or inability to use the electronic component package or book, even if Springer Science+Business Media, LLC, or the author(s) has been advised of the possibility of such damages.